Patients Are People

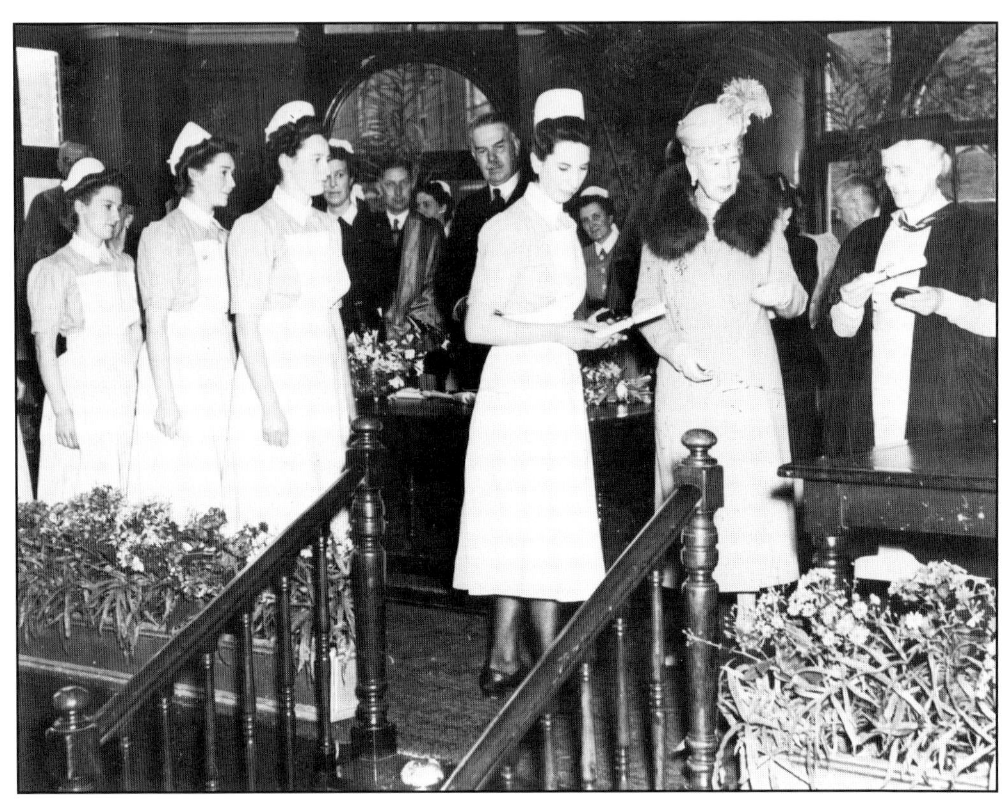

H M Queen Mary, President, later Patron, presents Certificates and Badges in the medical College Library 1946

FOREWORD

Perhaps the greatest compliment one can pay to a member of the staff of The London (or The Royal London as it is today) is to call him or her "a real Londoner". This Margaret Broadley most certainly is. She first joined The London in 1923 and in the years since then has been one of the leading figures in the life and folklore of the hospital. Today, in her Nineties, she has produced this book, a sequel to "Patients Come First", which brings her early story up to the present. It is a fascinating record of huge changes in nursing, with some valuable messages for today.

I had the great privilege of being Chairman of the Board of Governors of The London for some years until the Boards of all undergraduate teaching hospitals were abolished in 1974. During those years, I came to know that The London's reputation for pre-eminence in nursing (amongst other things) was well justified: and that people like Miss Broadley were responsible for it. It is a marvellous tradition: and I often recall one of Lord Evans' splendid remarks to his students to the effect that medical care counted for much less than nursing care. They both count, of course, but I know what he meant.

During these years the load on nurses has increased enormously, and today they have much less time than in the past to spend with the patient. Medical care today is immeasurably better: but sadly the personal bond between nurse and patient is almost certainly less close than in the past, and in this I feel we have lost something of crucial value. But in spite of that, I am staggered by the fact that the essential caritas of nursing still survives intact. Long may it do so.

We must all be very grateful to Margaret Broadley for her latest book. It records a period of unprecedented change in society generally, and consequently in nursing, from a very personal viewpoint. One can see why she became such a loved and respected figure at The London.

Harry Moore

Previous publications

Bandaging made easy. Faber & Faber
Sixth edition. Revised, 1943

Modern Living. Nursing & Community Service
Longmans Green & Co Ltd. 1968

Patients come first. Produced for The London Hospital Special Trustees
by Pitman Medical Ltd. 1980

ACKNOWLEDGEMENTS

My warmest thanks to all the London Hospital nurses who have contributed their experiences, vital to the text. I thank my nephew, Nicholas Hagger, for introducing me to modern methods and Malcolm Bell for his subsequent patience and forbearance.

I am grateful to Claire Daunton, former archivist, for her help and encouragement and to Jonathan Evans, archivist, for his unstinting help with photographs and access to records.

I am most grateful to Dame Phyllis Friend and Miss Peggy Nuttall who have given so generously of their time, specialised knowledge and expertise.

Finally, my grateful thanks for Sir Harry Moore at whose suggestion this book was written.

CONTENTS

CHAPTER ONE

THE EXODUS

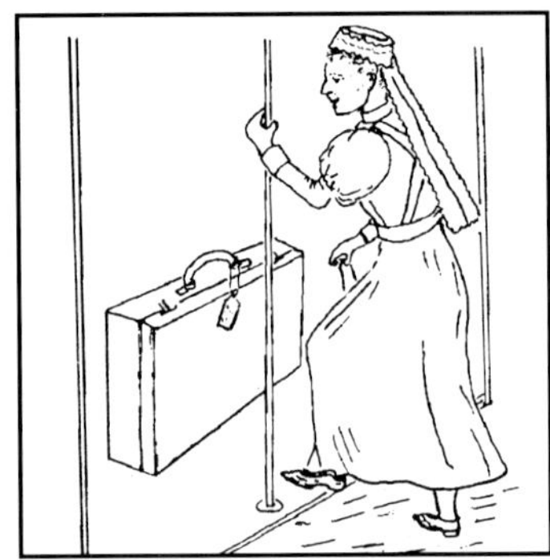

War was declared at 11 o'clock on Sunday morning, September 3rd 1939, but for the Nursing Staff at The London Hospital it began on Friday September 1st at 8 o'clock in the evening - in the first floor dining room. Sisters' dinner had been served as usual at 7pm, each Sister's individual napkin ring marking her place, menu cards on the table. The Senior Home Sister said grace, everybody sat and uniformed maids began serving - for many it was the last such meal they would eat in the dining room.

'The London' at that time, with nine hundred beds, was the largest voluntary hospital under one roof in the country. The Nursing Staff, including the 'Private Staff', was over seven hundred, of whom not one was married. It was 'The London's' proud boast that every nurse had a single room and of course they were all resident. The Nursing Staff was completely inbred. Nobody trained elsewhere was ever appointed to the staff and nobody who had left was allowed to return. Miss Lückes, Matron 1880 - 1919, considered that no examination devised by the State could compare with 'The London's' own certificate. In the twenties, State Registration, if not actively opposed, was not encouraged and nurses who wished to register did so without any help. Miss Reynolds, Matron since 1938, was doing her best to expedite it, but there was still a number of Sisters and Private Staff Nurses who had yet to register.

Whitechapel was predominantly a white area. Both the Albert Dock Seaman's and Poplar Hospitals lay between 'The London' and the docks. The first time I encountered a black patient was during my second night duty, in the second year of my training. With very rare exceptions the nursing staff were all white and I fancy the Swiss girl I took to the police station the following Monday to register as an alien was the only foreigner amongst us. 'The London's' Private Nursing Staff was unique and, from the time of

King Edward VII's emergency surgery on the eve of his Coronation, nursed everybody from Royalty downwards, in Europe as well as throughout England. Several Private Nurses had been in the Services during the 1914 - 1918 war; this was regarded as secondment, not leaving and they were valuable on the outbreak of another war.

Much publicity has been given to the subject of the evacuation of London's children. The children, accompanied by their teachers, needed homes and classroom space, but evacuation of London's teaching hospitals must have been a mammoth task. On the one hand, beds had to be available for the patients currently in the hospitals and service casualties as well as unknown numbers of victims of air raids and gas attacks. On the other hand, doctors and nurses were needed as never before and their training must be continued.

In the summer of 1939 I had attended a course of lectures on gas warfare. At one session the lecturer told us - there had been a massive gas attack leaving hundreds of casualties - what building in our immediate vicinity could be improvised to cope? A few minutes discussion left us thinking that the local Woolworth's would have to suffice. I saw myself - alone - all available floor space covered with semi-conscious victims - the mind boggled, but I am inclined to think that the people who planned the evacuation must have foreseen such eventualities.

On the eve of the N.H.S., in 1948, it was estimated that England had over five hundred hospitals with less than one hundred beds, of these over half had less than thirty. East Grinstead, for example, in the '20's, with a population of five to six thousand had a cottage hospital with twelve beds, one cot and an operating theatre; a workhouse infirmary with probably about the same number and an isolation hospital presumably able to take up to twenty in an epidemic. In the '30's the people of East Grinstead raised the money for a new hospital. They built imaginatively on the outskirts of the town, on a site with plenty of available land for extension. It had a men's and a women's ward, six cots, six private beds and an excellent theatre. One of my sisters had her appendix out in the old one, and the other, just before the war, her tonsils removed in the new. Having seen it, I could understand it becoming one of the most famous burns units in the country, but the vast majority of all these little hospitals were useless for evacuation. That left the mental and municipal hospitals. The Victorians built the mental hospitals as vast custodial institutions set in extensive grounds. The control of these had passed to the local authorities and they could make room both to nurse casualties and house nursing and medical staffs. Many municipal hospitals had begun life as workhouse infirmaries, some of them, too, had room for expansion and had the added advantage that they were already nursing the sick.

An Emergency Medical Service had been set up. London and the surrounding country was divided into ten sectors radiating from Charing Cross, with management control based on the larger voluntary/teaching hospitals. 'The London' was allocated Sectors I and II which covered the east and north east of London and parts of Essex, Herts and Middlesex, subdivided into fourteen units. A skeleton staff would remain at 'The London' to deal with the disposal of the remaining patients and receive the expected casualties. Everybody else was to be evacuated.

This must have required much thought on the part of Matron and her staff. Each unit required a Sister-in-charge, Sisters, Staff Nurses, first, second and third year student nurses. Training, academic as well as practical, must continue. There were just two qualified tutors, Miss Annie Harris and myself, we had both been qualified for one year, but there the similarityended. Annie, a teacher who had come into nursing late, qualified as a tutor on the minimum nursing experience - she was an academic and a brilliant organiser. I had embarked on the Tutor Course thinking how much better a Ward Sister I should be subsequently. One of the Sisters allocated to each unit was called 'Sister Tutor' and was to be responsible for some academic supervision of the student nurses. The consultants at the various units, whether they had, or not, previously given nursing lectures did so. Some combined classes of nurses and medical students. When we were summoned to the Dining Room, it had been cleared and rearranged. Fourteen tables manned by Sisters had been set up in the Dining Room, each with a pile of labels in a different colour. Evacuation by double decker bus would start by 9 o'clock the next morning - each could take one suitcase which she must be able to carry. My own destination was Warley Woods.

No tribute can be high enough for all the young people who trained during the war. Pre-war training was hard, but sheltered. In the wards, from the beginning the trainee was learning to accept responsibility. Off duty, she was hemmed in with petty restrictions. The Nurses' Homes were run much like the boarding side of a residential school. There was a boot rack on every floor where, in theory, a boot boy cleaned shoes. Home Sisters supervised closely - every nurse must leave her bed stripped and her window open when she went on duty - and lights out at 10:30 was rigorously enforced. It was, however, a way of life - everybody knew the rules. Suddenly - it was shattered - for ever.

The Matron greeting the arrivals at one unit stressed that she would not have Medical Students running in and out of the nurses' rooms. A friend of mine in that group had only recently been severely reprimanded by Home Sister - she had taken her own father to see her newly acquired Sister's 'bed sitting room' - to think of entertaining medical students there was beyond the wildest flights of fancy.

A number of these early evacuees have contributed towards the following early impressions.

The **West Ham Mental Hospital, Goodmayes**, distinguished by yellow labels, was the shortest distance away.

Violet Howlett (Mrs Haylett) writes:-

When my turn arrived to get on my friends and I hurried to the top deck and onto the front seat to get a good view of our journey. We were all in full indoor uniform. It was unheard of to wear it away from the wards, which added to the unusual situation. I had never been near a mental hospital and had no idea where Goodmayes was; it was disappointing to find it was hardly in the country at all and only took half an hour to get there. On arrival we were very apprehensive to see a group of very scruffy youths lounging against the entrance of the grim, grey building of the mental hospital. We assumed they were some of the patients we had noticed about the grounds as we drove in. Rather than risk being attacked, we all decided to stay put until they moved off. After a while one of the Sisters called up "Hurry up, come down, nurses, we have arrived". We replied that we couldn't until those men moved away. "Why not?" she inquired, and we explained about the 'patients', to which she replied. "Don't be so silly nurses, they are our own Medical Students". It was a group of sheepish nurses who then descended and hurried into the building.

Marjorie Rogers writes:-

My most vivid recollection is of the butterflies on the flowers in the grounds. I wondered why humans become embroiled in so many difficulties!

F Elizabeth Williams writes:-

The first or second night, when drinking tea in my bedroom with friends, there was a terrible noise outside and we decided the war had started in earnest - it was a heavy thunderstorm. The bedrooms had obviously been occupied by patients, the 'ablutions room' was fitted with keys to the taps. Everywhere was blacked out and all the paint work was very dark green. This was one of six bedrooms I occupied in this sprawling complex of buildings.

Dr Donald Hunter was the senior physician and Miss Phyllis Stanley Sister in charge. In the absence of patients, with all the emergency beds prepared for admission, all the splints padded and, for some strange reason, the draw sheets stitched by hand, we were informed that lectures would take place every morning. Dr Hunter and the Medical Superintendent, Dr Larkin, decided there were possibly some among the hospital's own patients who could benefit from medical treatment. Prof. William Ibbotson, Ear Nose and Throat Surgeon from the Prince of Wales Hospital, something of an eccentric, wearing an enormous black hat and cape, arrived daily in his pony and trap. The pony was tethered and put to grass during the time 'Ibby', as he became affectionately known, was working. From him, working in the wards, theatre and out patients, we gained continuity in this specialised field.

Gradually medical and surgical patients were admitted and the theatre became busy. One memorable morning when a number of patients in Female Ward One were prepared for operation, Mr Charles Donald, coming to do his round, found problems - somebody had allowed the paperboy into the ward - it was the fall of Dunkirk - no operations that day!

Air-raid casualties were admitted, mostly those with extensive burns. We used the RAF technique of floating the injured limb in a bag of saline. One patient remains in my memory, Jimmy aged seventeen. His legs were a charred mass. When the strip dressings were removed his constant cry, in true Cockney 'Gi' me a Tizer'. No doubt today's request in similar distress would be for a 'Coke'.

For those of us living long distances from home, days off were mostly spent taking long cycle rides into the Essex countryside. On one occasion Phyllis Baker and I cycled to Southend-on-Sea and back. We were badly sunburnt and found our uniform sleeves agony to wear. Walking from the hospital soon brought us to footpaths and country lanes. We often watched the dog fights' between the RAF and enemy planes. We were given the use of the patients' large concert hall for use after duty. With the loan of an old gramophone and records we spent many evenings dancing with the medical students. Professor Ibbotson would sometimes come to the concert hall, not to dance, but to play fugues. One or two people brought their violins. Along with the frequent need to don tin hats and man the stirrup pumps life was never dull.

Two events at Goodmayes remain very clear. The day an incendiary bomb reduced my bedroom to charred timbers and a sodden mass of plaster. It was not so much the loss of clothing etc., which caused distress, but the sight of my text-books, note-books and precious White Book (individual training record). The second book with the words written by Miss Annie Harris, '1st Book damaged by enemy action (2.5.41)' never really meant the same.

The second event took place in what had been the Craft Centre for the mental patients. This single storey building, situated some distance from the hospital and Nurses Home, became the communal bedroom for twelve of us. With beds and lockers tightly packed around the walls, large centre table, ablutions with horse-box doors, a kettle and a small electric fire we decided Craft Centre was an inappropriate name. We put a large notice, 'The Better Ole' on the door. Christmas was coming. We decided a party was called for. Letters were sent home for food of any kind. Large boxes arrived. We sent invitations to all the Sisters, concluding with 'Bring your own mug'. They came. It was a good party, those bleak winter days in the 'Better Ole' can never be forgotten.

Essex County Council Hospital & Workhouse, Orsett near Grays, Essex was the destination of the first of the evacuees.

Helen Walton writes:-

We left The London Hospital about midday on Friday September 1st on a double-decker bus. Dr William Evans was the Physician-in-charge, the surgeon came from the Dreadnought Hospital, Greenwich., Miss Laker was the Sister-in-charge. I was sent to empty wards which had to be prepared for the influx of expected air-raid casualties. I remember the air raid warning on the Sunday morning, after listening to the Prime Minister of course we expected casualties to appear immediately. The wards were full of elderly people and the nursing was shocking to us straight from 'The London'. Dr Evans set about transforming this regime, instead of being left to languish in bed, patients were dressed and encouraged to move about. This was the foundation of Modern Geriatric care and many years later as a Health Visitor on a Refresher Course one of the lecturers was Dr Couzens who had been the Medical Superintendent at Orsett and had followed in Dr Evans' footsteps. I was intrigued to meet this figure from my past. Some good did come out of the evacuation of London Hospital staff to Orsett.

Florence Chester (Mrs Walker) left 'The London' on the morning of Sunday, September 3rd - one of the second contingent. She writes:-

En route we picked up some staff from a Dr Barnardo's Home somewhere in Essex. During the journey we were surprised to see barrage balloons and then to hear the wail of the sirens for the very first time. War had been declared.

We arrived at lunch time, when we were welcomed and given a nice meal set at a very long table in the dismal dining room. After lunch we were shown to our quarters in a shoddy type of modern building - the rooms were quite nice although very sparse.

Next day I was introduced to Ward I, a downstairs ward in the old workhouse building, it was full of closely packed beds occupied by poor elderly male patients, many in cots and in the final stages of their lives. The nursing care was horrendous - there were pressure sores, sore mouths, and incontinence and only a minimum of attendance, this was not the sort of scene that I was used to and I felt upset by it. Within a few days these patients were transferred elsewhere and the ward was prepared for casualty intake.

Ward 1 became the reception area for army personnel with medical problems. The equipment was not up to 'London' standards but was adequate. This ward even had a padded cell complete with a strait jacket - the windows of the ward were sandbagged half way up cutting out a lot of natural light. The staff on the ward were at first mixed, some who were Irish girls lived in the village - they were from an agency and mostly auxiliary grade. The Ward Sister and Staff Nurse resented our intrusion in an obvious manner.

Gradually patients were admitted, some quite ill, some minor complaints and some with psychiatric problems often caused by the sudden shock of call-up and the fear of the unknown, there were also those who invented symptoms to effect a medical discharge.

After a week or two I was put on night duty. As a senior probationer in the second half of my third year, I was in charge of Ward 1 with a junior nurse, Susie Underwood. The darkness of the place, the cockroaches and field mice scurrying about, and the noises of night owls were terrifying. The ward was quite busy but it was still nice to see the dawn.

Belonging to the last century, - parts were very old, including a reception area where vagrants and homeless people came to shelter. They were given a bed and meals but, according to their age and stature, had to do work in return. On the ward was a list of food allowance according to age, height and health.

Dr Evans' lectures were always interesting, with his wry sense of Welsh humour. One notable instance was the occasion of a lecture on endocrine diseases, he showed slides and passed round photographs - asking for diagnoses and opinions. One such photograph of a small boy gave him many answers. As we shared lectures with medical students, one can imagine the amazement when Rachael White boldly suggested the child looked normal. 'Thank you nurse,' said he, 'that is myself aged five!' Much understanding of geriatric situations and endocrinology must have been gained by Dr Evans' studies at Orsett.

Off duty was a problem as there was so little to do. Most of the area was guarded by Army or A.R.P. personnel who were amazed to see our 'London' uniforms and there was a lot of interest and admiration. There were many orchards in the area and we were never short of gifts of plums and apples.

At the hospital security was also in evidence, on leaving or returning we had to check in at the gatehouse. A humorous incident occurred when one of our nurses going for a cycle ride on her day off was stopped by a military guard. She had no means of identification and was taken to the guardroom where a scrawled notebook fell under scrutiny. It contained lists, for example:

(7) I or II (5) II (3) J & C (4) Nil etc.

these were dinner lists! We hoped they enjoyed the joke as much as we did.
(For the uninitiated
I = full diet e.g. Meat.
II = Light e.g. fish.
J & C = Jelly and custard.)

The only social function I remember was a dance run by officers of the local command. A patient in the ward sent us each a corsage of carnations. We were told we must wear uniform, but surprise, surprise, only the Londoners did so, the others were allowed to wear their finery. Another example of 'Them and Us'.

Helen Paxton, (Mrs Harbeck) recalls:-

Orsett was a small one street English village with very little traffic. There was a weekly bus to London, so all the nurses used bicycles. Madge Booth (Neé Hungerford) and I were billeted at the Old Vicarage where the elderly Vicar insisted on us attending evening prayers in the kitchen. Madge and I worked on the men's surgical ward, where for the first time in my life I met young soldiers who teased blushing probationers wearing new uniforms!.

In the following months during the Battle of Britain, we often watched aerial battles over the flat farmland - sometimes a wounded German pilot was admitted to a side ward, guarded by Local Defence Volunteers.

The Tipper Twins (Barbara Miller and Jean Caddick) were transferred from Warley Woods just before Christmas 1939. Barbara died in April 1994; during her long illness she and her sister made notes about the time they spent at Orsett, kindly sent by her husband Dr. R Mac Miller .

The Nursing Staff made us very welcome and together we started, under the direction of an Orthopaedic Surgeon from the nearby Albert Dock Hospital, an active programme of getting many of these patients out of bed and on to chairs or Zimmers in an effort to teach them to walk again. As a result of this and the admission of patients from local Anti-Aircraft batteries and Searchlight units, we became very busy. (The army patients soon began to look on the hospital as a hotel compared with their usual quarters and were very loath to leave!)

Our first winter was a very severe one. Most of us were billeted in an old Rectory some way from the hospital, so a rickety old ambulance used to collect us in the mornings and return us at night - until a particularly heavy fall of snow made the journey impossible and the ambulance could not get through. Joy of joys, an empty ward with full central heating was opened up for us and we spent a very happy week gradually getting thawed out - it was bliss compared with the cold, damp Rectory, where, when we put hot-water bottles in our beds, the steam began to rise.

In time we took over more of the wards and the Geriatric and long-stay patients became separated from those with acute medical and surgical conditions, so we drifted apart from the original Orsett Staff, who I think became a little in awe of us all. We look on our stay there as an extremely happy time and would not have missed it for the world.

St Margaret's Hospital and Workhouse, Essex County Council.

Peggy Shaul (Mrs Freeman) writes:-

Miss Freda Hall, (Mrs Taylor), and Miss Johnston were in charge. They were both known as "Old Dragons" at the London Hospital, but no one could have been kinder to us. Miss Hall was known as "Dear Freda" and Miss Johnston as "Fanny" - between ourselves, of course! In our youth we felt very superior since we were London Hospital Nurses - my time there was very happy. We were in makeshift dormitories with very basic equipment - but we had fun.

We were packing dressing drums when Sister came in and announced "Nurses, war has been declared" - but still we had no real idea of what war entailed. I worked in the Reception Room, and saw my first and only case of tetanus, a man, who was admitted to the wards and died. I helped nurse my first case of cerebro-spinal meningitis, the patient recovered, which in those days was quite an achievement, and I remember we were congratulated on our nursing, - being very junior I was really thrilled about the whole experience.

I also helped in the Dental Department where Mr Herman was the Dental Surgeon - there were three dental students and Barbara Allen and myself to assist. In their spare time the students together with Barbara Allen - violin - and Betty Boase - cello - formed a small band. I remember these things from photographs and autographs of that time, all very tattered, on which I have written "Rescued from the Blitz, 1940". A number of our patients were from the Essex Yeomanry who were stationed nearby. I spent Christmas 1939 at Epping and was at The London Hospital when the Blitz started, my room being amongst those bombed at a very early stage - by Christmas 1940 I was at Chase Farm Hospital, Enfield - there we had Miss Young, who hauled me over the coals for having an untidy ward!! "No matter how busy you are nurse, you always clear up as you go along!" Advice which has stood me in good stead all through my nursing life. I am forever grateful to her.

Essex County Council Hospital and Workhouse, Billericay.

Jessie Edwards, (Mrs Frost), was one of the group whose departure was delayed until the Sunday. She writes:-

The siren started as we arrived and were walking down the drive! We were all told to lie down where we were. This was not funny as we were in uniform. It was also a false alarm but it was a very grubby lot of nurses who reported to the hospital. I and another nurse were billeted with an elderly lady and her daughter Marjorie. They were very nice and employed a domestic help, who, later, was to drive the milk cart. The house, situated the outskirts of a large wood was lovely and the garden was delightful. It was heaven to me, but not easy for them coping with two nurses especially when we were on night duty.

Huts, to be used as wards, were quickly erected in the hospital grounds and the elderly who were cared for in the main building were either sent home or to other institutions. The hospital was run by a Master and Matron and it could not have been easy for them to be suddenly taken over by so many new staff. Some of the elderly had to remain and they were taught air-raid drill. It was a pathetic sight to see them trying to get under the bed clutching a pillow. We, also, had to lie under the bed with the patients. I remember on one of these occasions as we lay under the bed one elderly gentleman wanted to go to the toilet, but he could not wait and seeing the open window he aimed straight through it. We settled in very quickly and acute cases were admitted, the huts were mainly for soldiers, and these were filled with both medical and surgical cases. As the war continued we regularly heard the siren. At about 7 o'clock every evening, we would hear the German bombers, who always seemed to be heading for London, flying overhead. In spite of continual aerial activity, life was good. I was very happy with Marjorie and her mother. Marjorie taught me to drive the car and lots of other things.

The operating theatre was very small having only an anaesthetic room, an operating room and a sterilising room. All the windows were blackened and bricked on the outside. The theatre was in constant use. While I was Theatre Nurse all the lights failed, including the emergency ones. The surgeon was in the middle of a major operation, it was pitch black inside but the sun was shining outside. One of the doctors had a brainwave, Why not use the sun?'. So the table was moved to the door of the sterilising room, a stainless steel tray was propped up on the steriliser, a student held another tray above the operation site and with the reflection of the sun on these two trays the operation was completed. The patient made a good recovery and she did not hear of the excitement that had taken place.

We had good experience in the medical, surgical and children's wards, we had to attend lectures regularly and there was a lot of studying to be done.

The wards filled quickly. The soldiers' wards were heated by large closed-in stoves in the middle of the wards, and these had to be continually stoked. It was a dirty chore but if they were neglected they would go out and they were difficult to light. One day when I was on duty in one of these wards the house surgeon came in and asked me to close the door. He commanded silence and then said, Some of you boys are shamming, and I know who you are, I will give you until the morning to sort yourselves out'. Sure enough half the ward decided they were fit enough to be discharged, and they returned to their unit. I felt sorry for them for who knows what the future held for them. We saw many 'dog fights', as they were called during the daylight raids in the summer of 1940. We should not have watched but it was fascinating seeing the Spitfires (the name given to the little fighter planes) weaving in and out of the flying bombers shooting down some. I did see a Spitfire shot down and as the pilot parachuted out, the German plane followed him and shot at him. When he was admitted he had a bullet through his heel lodging in his big toe. He was lucky not to have been killed. He asked before his operation, 'could he please have the bullet because he would like to return it'.

Hertfordshire County Council Workhouse and Hospital, Hitchen.

Susan Grace (Mrs Rooze) writes:-

The block, which had been left for us, was apart from the other buildings. On going round we found one poor old lady who had been left there by mistake! I was put on night duty, and we spent the time cleaning lockers, making up beds, teasing tow and padding endless splints. We also made gangee jackets and hundreds of theatre swabs.

The Matron seemed to be very domineering and insisted that we got up at tea time for our lectures so that her daughter who was still at school could attend them. After a time when none of the expected casualties appeared we were sent to work in the wards. These were awful - very low beds, terribly close together, and we spent all night changing incontinent patients and trying to get the 'wanderers' back to bed. Many of the patients were epileptic, which was pretty frightening at first. We also had to go down to the cells to dress any wounds that the tramps might have. These were usually burns from falling asleep too near their fires. Drunken soldiers were also put down there but they were under guard, so even if they had injuries there was a soldier with us.

Our food was put into a cupboard which was infested with cockroaches, but in spite of all this we were quite happy and everybody was marvellous, especially dear Miss McCreath who understood how depressing it was.

At the beginning we had to share rooms and since I was on night duty and the other girl was on day duty we didn't see much of each other. I was there about six months mostly on night duty and was very glad to be sent back to The London Hospital. I spent a year as Staff Nurse Queen Mary at Brentwood and after that went to The Croft Home at Reigate for a time - that was lovely for me as I had started nursing there in 1938 before coming to Hospital and knew Miss Jordan the Matron very well. I was also sent to Haileybury College for several weeks.

'Brentwood' here refers to The London Hospital Annexe at Brentwood, a hutted hospital rented by 'The London'. Patients were admitted directly to it or transferred from Whitechapel. Here they were nursed by London Hospital nurses and looked after by London Hospital doctors, gradually withdrawn from the Sector Hospitals.

'The Croft Home' was a small London Hospital Annexe at Reigate, opened in the 1920s for women patients. As pre-nursing students girls accepted for training at 'The London' spent up to a year there until they were old enough to take up their vacancies.

Chase Farm Hospital, Enfield - Middlesex County Council -

F Elizabeth Williams writes in 1941.

Daphne Elliott and I arrived together and were greeted by Miss Billington, Sister-in-charge. As there was no room for us in the Nurses Home we were to be billeted out. We were accompanied to a house about a mile away where the lady said that she was ill and could not take us. She had been in touch with a fairly near neighbour who happened to be the Cemetery Keeper. He and his wife, Mr & Mrs Gambles, lived at Cemetery Lodge and this is where we lived. They were a warm hearted couple, made us feel welcome and would share their milk ration with us at bedtime. All meals were taken at the hospital. So that we could get in when they were out, Mr Gamble gave us a front door key. (I never saw a back door, presumably this led out to the cemetery). Daphne and I arranged always to leave the key under the nearest grave stone, just inside the huge iron gates! The system worked well - our bicycles were useful between 'home' and the hospital. It was a severe winter, I remember skidding and falling off my bicycle on the icy roads!

I was glad to be in the ward of Miss Constance Fuller, who had been Sister Turner. Turner had been my second ward. I shall always remember Miss Fuller for her wonderful nursing care of her patients.

Ward progress reports, which each nurse had to read and sign, were introduced about then. I felt less shocked by this new experience after discussing on one point on which I disagreed.

Like that of the nurses, the training of other students was disrupted.

Miss Peggy Nuttall, who was at home on September 3rd, writes:-

War was declared on a most lovely autumn morning, a Sunday. The sky was blue and cloudless, as it had been all summer and it was warm, blissfully warm. For nearly a year we had lived in the shadow of war. Mr Chamberlain's telegram hadn't stopped the sandbags being filled or the blackout material bought together with the candles and torches. Little brown cardboard boxes held gas masks, but one or two important people were known to posses tin hats. So it was a lively awareness of war - because of Little Poland - that made us all switch on our wirelesses just before 11 o'clock. In his rather prim precise voice the Prime Minister told us that his telegram had been unanswered and that, consequently, we were at war with Germany. But what galvanised - or petrified - those of us in London was to hear, just after big Ben had struck on the wireless the wail of sirens: an air-raid alert. Some people expected to be killed within minutes by bombs dropped by enemy aircraft (we were to wait for nearly twelve months for those bombs to come raining down onto Mile End Road one Saturday afternoon). But in September 1939 no-one knew what to expect. Fortunately the 'All-clear' sounded almost immediately and, surprisingly, we were all still alive. More than fifty years later no doubt this sounds silly, but many can testify to its truth.

My mother went into the kitchen to get on with the Sunday joint. My father, ever inquiring and inquisitive, went out into the road to gaze up into the skies and talk to the neighbours. My brother and I merely looked at each other. I was a final year student of massage, medical gymnastics and electrotherapy at the new School of Physical Medicine in Turner Street, a new annexe of The London Hospital's old Out Patients Department. We had been told to report for duty at the outbreak of war. I suspect we were all an added burden to the overworked Matron's Office. We had been warned of the possibility of evacuation - another word which had acquired a totally new meaning when little school children with labels and gas masks and expectant mothers with pink forms (this was an official description) were packed off in their hundreds from all main line st tions with trains going North and West. The South Coast was to be out of bounds for the duration.

I packed a small bag and caught a Green Line coach to Whitechapel. After reporting to Matron's Office where they were still clipping the corners off notes, I spent the night in the Cavell Home but the next few days are a total blank and I next remember going to Chase Farm Hospital to be greeted by Miss Billington - or 'The Bill' as she was known when she was out of earshot. On reflection, after all these years, what a nuisance we must have been. Nobody knew what was happening, when the hostilities would start - or what to do with a hoard of young, able-bodied women who, although 'willing' hadn't even the embryonic skills of probationers. After a few days we 'helped' in the wards with the few remaining patients who seemed to be too ill, or too old, to have been moved. In one ward I found myself allowed to help with last offices of an elderly patient and I remember reflecting that this was an odd war.

Between times at Chase Farm we sat in the sun (quaintly rolling bandages which seemed to have occupied so much time in the 1st World War) and improved our suntans. Some of us were lodged in nearby houses others slept in dormitories. We must have been a great nuisance to those in authority. We were all willing, not particularly able and there was really nothing for us to do. I have no recollection of how, or when we returned to The London, but we did, and took our finals while the phoney war was waged at home and the real war took place in the Atlantic and the North Sea. I finished my training in 1940, passed and went to work at St. George-in-the-East in Wapping, and that is quite another story.

CHAPTER TWO

WARLEY WOODS

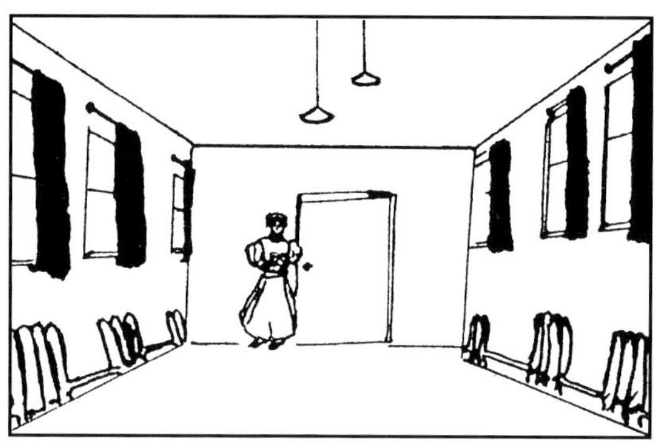

Warley Woods was a large mental hospital on the outskirts of Brentwood. As we drove in through the main entrance our first impression was of sprawling buildings scattered over extensive grounds. From the main building we were directed on to the 'Admission Block'. This was a large, new building, which, with the exception of Dining and Recreation rooms and a number of single bedrooms to be used for trained staff, had been cleared in readiness for us. 'Cleared' was the operative word, black-out had been fitted at all windows otherwise it was completely empty. Had the bombing of London started on September 3rd the casualties sent to us would have been in a parlous plight. A block used for convalescent patients had been prepared for the nurses in training. 'The London's' boast was that every probationer had a single room. What awaited them were large dormitories - bed, chair, bed, chair, all round the walls.

Looking back, the upheaval for those in charge of all sector hospitals must have been enormous. They were probably as apprehensive as we were. I cannot remember that we were welcomed, but we were soon provided with tea - in large enamel jugs already mixed with milk and sugar!

The Sister in charge of our unit was a senior private Staff Nurse, Miss Nellie Ball, who had been in the Army in the last war. Mr Alan Perry, the senior surgeon, was also a war veteran. Doctor Horace (later Lord) Evans was our physician and there was another surgeon from elsewhere. 'Thc Horace Evans's and the other surgeon and his wife had taken houses nearby - outside the hospital. Mr Alan Perry and his wife, herself a Londoner and a marvellous voluntary helper and their excellent maid, Ethel, had accommodation somewhere in the hospital.

Throughout the war the way in which the nurses in training accepted everything that happened never ceased to amaze me, they just cheerfully carried on. We were all to eat together. It was disconcerting as we assembled for breakfast next morning to find that we had been supplied with one portion of egg and bacon, six of bacon and tomato, with bacon and fried potatoes for the rest. Admittedly at 'The London', the food of Sisters and nurses was not the same, but their meals were at different times. Eating together, such distinction was distasteful. Later, we gathered round our one radio and heard the official declaration of war. The subsequent brief air-raid warning made no impact.

One bus load postponed from the Saturday arrived at their destination just as the siren went. Matron interrupted her welcome to say 'Lie down'. Thought better of it and yelled, 'SCATTER - I don't want all my nurses killed at once.' My sister was spending the weekend with my mother, and they were in Church when the siren went. Thinking only of her three month old son, asleep in his pram in the garden - resident help was common in 1939 - my sister ran for home thus unwittingly heading a stampede emptying the Church in seconds.

The all important question was how do you occupy fifty to sixty young women, when there is nothing to do and nothing to do it with. Nellie Ball was in favour of strict discipline. Mr Perry said the young people would lose a lot of time off when things got going, give them as much as possible now. I knew that the next State Examinations were only a month away. The June results had not been good so, as I was one of the only two qualified Nurse Tutors, our contingent contained a number of re-entries. I regarded this lull as a heaven-sent opportunity. Actually, teaching was about the only thing we could do; both Mr Perry and Dr Evans were willing to help, so we started straight away on intensive coaching for all nurses in training.

Within a few days furniture and equipment began to arrive, their unpacking, sorting and disposal produced some work and by degrees it was possible to include practical projects in our teaching programme. Our efforts paid off, not only were the results good but it was the only time in the whole of my teaching experience that Matron's Office at 'The London' received a letter of commendation from the General Nursing Council!

Kathleen Mortimer (Mrs Mizen) was also at Warley. Presumably she was not a State Examination candidate, she does not even mention that side of her training! She writes:-

We filled both the upstairs and downstairs of Woodside Villa, which was immediately named 'Woodbine Willie'. A trench was dug just outside for us - later - to stand and shiver in during Air Raids, which were mostly at night. One late evening we crowded round the door waiting and waiting to go out - eventually Home Sister came down the stairs saying, 'I am sorry to have been so long but I refuse to be bombed without my corsets on!' These night-time excursions soon ceased and another plan was executed. When the siren sounded the upstairs contingent would come down and share our beds. My friend said to me, 'You pop in with me, one never knows what might be descending on us!'

Meals were quite an ordeal - there were enough spoons, knives and forks for only half of us. When you had finished your meal you dashed off, washed these up and handed them to the next one in the queue.

In the beginning, too, everybody trailed off to 'The London' with empty suitcases returning with more necessities or cherished possessions. The mental hospital authorities supplied us with food and all essential services. We were interested to find hospital deliveries were made by one member of staff, whether or not a trained nurse we did not know, supervising two or three able-bodied patients. The hospital was virtually a self supporting unit, there was a farm and big vegetable garden. The workshops made and repaired furniture, bedding, clothing and suchlike. We were told that apart from stamps and alcohol there was nothing they could not produce. All patients who could do so were seemingly happily engaged on suitable work.

At 'The London' there was virtually no social life, the mental authorities invited us to share theirs. Soon after our arrival we were asked to go to their monthly dance. I had no suitable mufti, but as May Perry was my size and would lend me a dress it was decided I should escort our nurses. In a 'Paul Jones' I picked up a male nurse. First time round he inquired, 'you're one of the girls from 'The London'. Hardly a girl, I said, 'yes'. Next time round he queried 'Do you like it here?' Again I answered, 'yes'. Third time he said, 'Pity you've such a bloody lot of Sisters with you!' I could think of nothing better to say than, 'yes' but I don't think I was ever the same again. That description couldn't fit me!

My youngest sister was married on the first Saturday of the war. Nellie Ball was doubtful about letting me go, but Mr Perry said he was going to town anyway and took me to London Bridge Station. The bridegroom was in the Territorials and had been given forty-eight hours leave, so on the Monday morning my sister, an electrical demonstrator, went to work as usual. The manager, when told of her marriage, said that the Electricity Company concerned did not employ married women and dismissed her forthwith! She was back home by mid morning.

At last, after about six weeks it was decided we could admit patients. We were told we should be receiving a consignment of soldiers from a nearby military hospital, evidently they were preparing for service casualties. Our patients were expected early in the afternoon. The wards were fully staffed, a suitable tea prepared, even the operating theatre was ready. Time went on, cocoa was substituted for tea, and eventually, about 7 o'clock in the evening, a bus drew up. From it tumbled twenty odd walking men in army uniform. They might have been the hard core of any medical ward, all obviously unfit for service overseas even if not the spectacular cases we anticipated. Kathleen Mortimer recalls "We were all agog and even excited! We felt quite guilty that we had hoped they would be casualties." We were however delighted to receive them and they fairly revelled in the attention bestowed on them.

Gradually, we began to admit patients whom we should normally have described as 'T.C.Is'. People who had been seen by a consultant and recommended for admission hence T for To, C for Come and I for In. It meant that the beds were occupied, the theatre was in use and work was proceeding. By Christmas we were settled into a routine and thanks to the efforts of May Perry everybody thoroughly enjoyed the festivities. There was a rash of engagements among the student nurses - an inevitable result of war.

The winter of 1939/40 was a severe one. The nurses, from their 'Villa', stumbled uncomplainingly through the snow. We began to realise just how much we had been cosseted. We came on duty one morning to find Lillie May, Night Sister, trying to deal with a flood from a burst pipe. Instead of the immediate response there would have been at 'The London' an urgent telephone call for a plumber elicited the reply that they were much too busy dealing with their own bursts to deal with ours. It was a Houseman who discovered where to turn the water off!

The nurses adapted themselves. **Kathleen Mortimer** continues:

We had a good hockey and tennis team and played with the doctors and medical students on the ground belonging to the Mental hospital. Occasionally we were invited to the Saturday night dances there to partner the patients. They sat on one side of the hall and we were on the other. As soon as the music piped up someone would grab you and pull you round the floor rather than dance. One such evening my partner said to me, 'I've been here eighteen months now, how long have you been here? It was sad to see children chained to their wardens as they could be dangerous.

During the latter part of our stay we had patients, both civilian and service casualties. By this time too we all had a bed to ourselves and enough knives and forks to go round. If it had been a boring part of our early training it was certainly not without amusement and happy times.

Warley Woods was probably unique among the Sector Hospitals in that we were in, but not of, the main hospital. As far as nursing was concerned we were in exactly the same situation as at 'The London'. The surroundings and equipment were different, but there was no outside influence.

We learned that other people did things differently. One day in the first week after the arrival of patients, the Ward Sisters discovered that the dinner sent consisted of big containers of soup - and pudding. They rang up the kitchen to say that the main course had been left out. The staff were apologetic and five minutes later there was another delivery - of soup. It had never occurred to us that one day a week the patients' main meal could be just soup and pudding. This was during the phoney war and before rationing had really started. We were amused to find that the British Army, or our part of it, shared our views!

So - what did the first six months of the war do for us? It had shaken our complacency. As trained staff we had begun to realise what a privileged life we had led. On duty, efficient backup services had ensured the smooth running of wards and departments. Off duty, we had hardly been aware that we were waited on hand and foot. On the other hand we were more free. It was ridiculous that trained nurses of many years standing were 'marked in' to breakfast like children arriving at school. The Nurses Homes were locked at ten o'clock at night, after which time we had to pick up a 'Leave of Absence Book' from Night Sister's office and tiptoe through a ward of sleeping patients to reach our rooms. For myself, I was happy at Warley Woods and not at all pleased when Matron told me that I was to move on to Haymeads.

Main building, Warley Hospital, Brentwood 1995

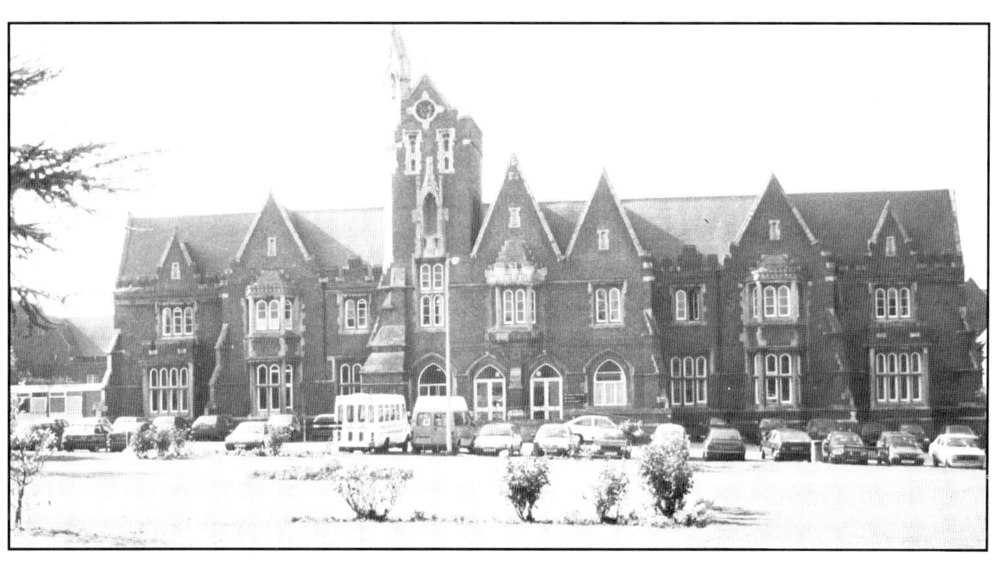

CHAPTER THREE

HAYMEADS

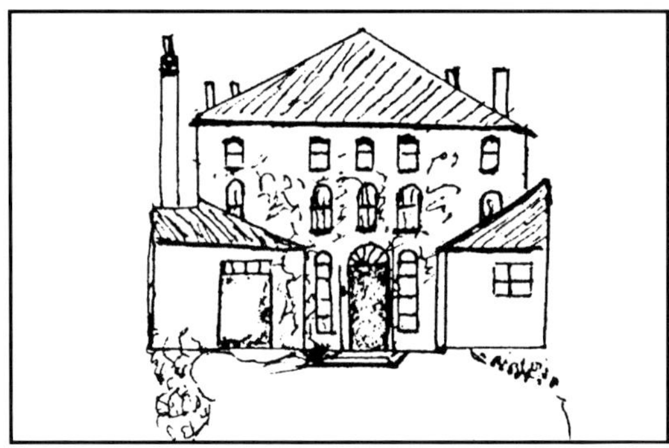

It was dark when I arrived at Haymeads in Bishop's Stortford. One of our young soldiers at Warley had been diagnosed as having cerebrospinal meningitis (spotted fever), and Dr Evans would not let me leave until he had received the report on my nose and throat swabs. That may have been why I was so late, but my first recollection of Haymeads is of wandering round the grounds in the blackout, looking for the entrance to the Nurses Home. I had been to the main building and been told there was no room in the Nurses Home, neither was there a billet available. For the night I was to sleep in a side ward off one of the wards. It was suggested perhaps I should have a bath in the Nurses Home first. In the Home I ran into Miss Leslie, Sister Buxton, the much loved 'Auntie B' who invited me to have a cup of tea. Another London Hospital Sister, Ruth Brackett, was there and a Ward Sister trained at U.C.H. (University College Hospital). I had spent a week in the course of my tutor training at U.C.H, I had my midday meal with their Sisters. Day by day they came in, buried their heads in their newspapers and ignored a stranger. The rudest lot of women I had ever met. The U.C.H Sister and I looked at one another with dislike. Nobody could have foreseen that we should become life long friends, or that I would be Godmother to her first baby. I came to regard her much as I did my youngest sister - she certainly had the same capacity for falling in and out of love.

I was glad on another count to meet a 'UCH' Sister. Constance Dobie (Lady Jameson) and I had gone there at our own request. 'UCH' had embarked on a totally new form of nurse education, 'The Block'. Instead of tired nurses leaving the wards at 8pm for lectures, their student nurses were taken, in smaller groups, right out of the wards for 2 or 3 weeks at a time. Constance and I knew the theory of it and had seen it at work. Now I could find out how a Ward Sister viewed it.

Haymeads was totally different from Warley. The latter was a well-established institution, where space had been made to accommodate victims of war emergency. Haymeads, on the other hand, had evolved as a result of definite policy. Doctor Balme, the medical superintendent, writing his first year's report, describes the situation. 'Should they expand as a mere improvisation to meet a temporary emergency or, taking advantage of the unique opportunity, attempt something more permanent'. The latter was the course that was taken. Haymeads was a hundred-year-old Public Assistance Institution built for workhouse inmates, casuals and the chronic infirm. It had, however, a newly opened modern Casual Department, a few good wards and a nursery block, from this an Emergency Hospital was created capable of receiving over eight thousand casualties in a crisis. To begin with nine units, built on the pavilion principle, connected by a covered way, an operation and X-ray block, kitchen and additional nurses' quarters were erected. A further eight were added later.

The provision of Nursing staff for a general hospital evolved so rapidly from a Poor Law Infirmary presented great difficulties. There were only a small number of trained nurses on the original staff. The Civil Nursing Reserve, a war time emergency body, could not have provided what was needed. The evacuees from the London hospitals, a cross section of their nursing staff, i.e. Sisters including Tutors, Staff Nurses and Probationers, was the answer. At the commencement of the war such a group of over fifty was transferred from the Prince of Wales Hospital, Tottenham. The Nurses Training School was thus established from the outset. A similar consignment from The London Hospital had followed later.

Haymeads had, however, one other great asset, the Master and Matron. Mrs Friend was not only unusually well qualified - she had even nursed in a small-pox unit - but was an outstandingly capable woman. She took each enlargement in her stride and won the respect and loyalty of all the motley assortment of trained nurses on her staff. Geriatric patients were the main occupants of the two wards in the original block. The Sisters in charge of them were widely experienced, they were not State Registered, it is doubtful whether they were even, in the accepted sense of the word, 'trained'. They understood old people. Every patient was given her full name and status - no slip shod 'dear' or Christian names - no tying up their hair with blue ribbon either, those who were up were meticulously dressed. Student nurses had much to learn there.

To quote again from Dr Balme's report:- 'The Ministry of Health having decided Haymeads should be one of the main paediatric centres for the sector, provision was made not only for the full use of the excellent nursery block, but also for the opening of special children's wards in the hospital. A considerable number of children suffering from a great variety of complaints had already been treated, and the transfer of Miss Leslie, Senior Sister of the Children's Department of The London Hospital, greatly helped in the organising of this department. An increasing number of sick children being transferred here from various London Hospitals, this department grew rapidly in size and importance.'

My 'UCH' friend, Gladys, had been the first Sister appointed to the emergency section. Her first job, in a completely bare hut, had been to list every item of equipment that a surgical ward required. As originally planned, each hut had forty beds, very close together. A hut was set aside for emergency use and when the Battle of Britain began, trained staff were on call at night on a rota system. Those of us living in billets, or at Plaw Hatch, slept there when on call, making sure there would be no delay should an emergency arise. The patients from the adjoining men's ward were in the habit of bringing early morning tea to those on call. What would Miss Luckes have said?

My memories of Haymeads fall into two distinct sections - work and play. As their tutor, it was important that I knew how all the student nurses, from both The London and Prince of Wales Hospitals, were faring. Matron had wisely decreed that I should, like the Ward Sisters, have alternate weekends off duty, so I spent my weekends working happily in the wards. The Sisters came from a wide variety of teaching Hospitals. I think we were all agreed that they, and their methods, were just as good as our own.

We found Haymeads Casual Ward fascinating. As children, playing in the garden on summer evenings, we were familiar with the enquiry of the occasional tramp, "Is this the way to the Union?". We knew the building in question as the 'workhouse'. The welfare of vagrants was of no interest to me then and at 'The London' our only contact with them was when the occasional emergency admission of one arose. However, Haymeads was different. My office overlooked the road passing the hospital. Sitting at my desk in the early evenings I could see any approaching tramps, or vagrants. Each one would stop nearby, empty his pockets, hide the contents in the hedge and come, completely destitute, to the hospital.

Back in the 19th Century a new Poor Law Act was introduced permitting the amalgamation of two or more Parishes in a Union, hence the term, Common Workhouse. The aim was to keep the rates as low as possible and the accommodation known as a casual ward was to be of a lower scale than that provided for paupers. Various poor laws had improved conditions and the vagrants of 1940 were given a bath, supper, bed and breakfast. Each was required to carry out such work, if any, as was required before being sent on his way with bread and cheese for his next meal. From the classroom one could hear sufficient of the bath, supervised by a porter, to decide whether that particular inmate was in favour of, or against, bathing. Haymeads was justly proud of their newly opened casual wards. In addition to ample accommodation for men there was room for ten women and children and special facilities for washing clothes. The Poor Law was abolished in 1930 and control of the workhouses and infirmaries passed to the Local Authorities, finally the National Assistance Act of 1948 destroyed its last vestiges. A vast range of benefits was introduced, replacing the casual ward.

To begin with local people welcomed nurses, rather than children, as evacuees into their homes. However, after the initial period of euphoria, nurses' hours, particularly night duty, were found to be difficult. An outbreak of measles and the subsequent fear of infection increased householders' reluctance to accept them, so the Ministry decided to accept the generous offer of Mrs Trevithick to place her residence Plaw Hatch Hall at their disposal. Dr Balme reported that sixty nurses could be accommodated there and it should prove a comfortable house for staff. It was first used temporarily, for the duration of one set only, by The London Hospital's Preliminary Training School. Mrs Hanbury wanted Hylands, her country home near Chelmsford, previously used in this capacity, for other purposes, and Merrymeade at Brentwood was not yet available.

When I arrived, Miss Annie Harris was in charge of 'The London's' student nurses and those from The Prince of Wales Hospital had their own Tutor. Both were to return and I was to take charge of the two groups. In theory that was simple - both were following the same syllabus and working for the same examinations. In practice, the two groups combined for doctors and other special lectures but the tutorial lines previously followed were so different I never tried to amalgamate them. In addition, from the staffing angle it was more convenient to have two smaller groups rather than one large one away from the wards at any time. Some of the students lived in the Haymeads Nurses' Home, some were billeted locally. The Prince of Wales Hospital was more missionary minded than The London Hospital and had a small number of non-white nurses in training. On one occasion, I took a couple of new arrivals to their billets. Bishops Stortford was in a rural area, the people who lived there would probably never have seen anybody other than white - certainly their prospective hostess had not. She opened the door, took one look at me and my two dark skinned companions and shut the door. My sympathies were divided equally. Surely somebody had blundered, the householder should have been warned.

I enjoyed teaching in a smaller and less formal environment. When I first went to 'The London' my father told me never to borrow or to lend money. He hadn't anticipated war. The student nurses were, like the rest of us, in strange surroundings in difficult times. I reckoned to keep a £20 float available for unexpected train fares and other auxiliary expenses. It was completely unofficial - and I always got it back.

Taking blood pressure had always previously been a medical procedure. Now it was to be done by the nursing staff. First we were to be instructed and then teach it. Teaching the Sisters proved highly entertaining and generally ended with some kind of joint medical nursing jaunt. To save fuel, clocks were put on two, instead of the customary one, hour, this double 'summer time' gave long light evenings. We explored the local country on foot, on bicycles or, if anybody had a little petrol, by car. We discovered a homely restaurant whose proprietress took pride in her cooking. Several of us were there one evening, the main course was rabbit. It struck me that my joint was a funny shape and singularly devoid of meat, but when we came to leave the proprietress told us that there was one rabbit joint still in the pot - the ham bone added for flavouring had gone! She insisted on charging for one meal less.

There was a certain amount of organised entertainment for Sisters as well as nurses. At Christmas Mrs Friend organised a coach trip to Cambridge - to the pantomime. When she asked the coach driver to stop he opened the door, evidently thinking as I did, that somebody was about to be sick, but no, Mrs Friend produced a hamper and, in the black-out,unearthed glasses of sherry to fortify us for the evening! A pantomime was high entertainment for me! My father, when I was considered too young to be included, once took my two brothers to a London pantomime. The younger one wept because Robinson Crusoe was a girl. Father was so put out that future visits were to Maskelyne and Cook at St. George's Hall - a pantomime was a new experience.

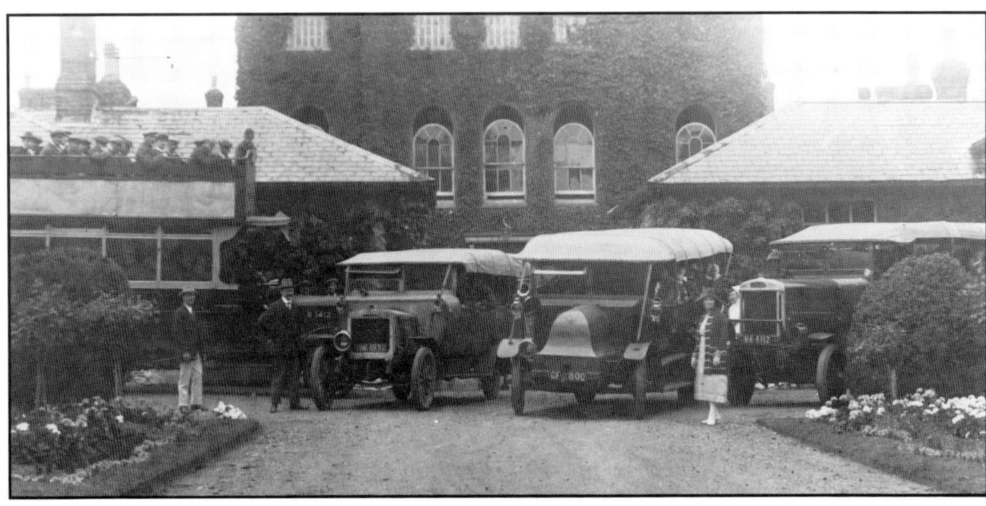

Double decker bus and char-a-banc assembled for inmates outing (late1920s)

I was billeted at first, together with Ruth Brackett, in a well to do family where Cook would leave our breakfast ready to cook for ourselves. With several other Sisters I spent some months in Plaw Hatch, where the chief disadvantage was an inadequate water supply. It was obviously not on the main and by the time the night nurses had had baths and gone on duty the water tanks were empty. We all carried quart bottles filled with water in the handle- bar baskets of our bicycles so we could at least clean our teeth. It was fun, but I was not sorry to be moved to the Nurses Home.

I had known Miss Leslie for a long time. She was essentially a casualty of the 1914-18 war and should have had a large family - instead she stood out as The London's foremost Children's Ward Sister, 'Auntie B', the legendary queen of Buxton Ward. I had worked in Buxton - twice, the first time I caught scarlet fever, the second, diphtheria, after which Matron, Miss Monk, said we would not bother with completing my children's experience! When I became Sister of Harrison, the adjoining ward, and her neighbour, my predecessor told me that she never borrowed from other wards. I gathered that the same could not be said of all. My very first day, as I served the patient's dinners I found a strange Ward maid, carrying two plates, at my elbow - Buxton was two dinners short. The Haymeads authorities appreciated her magical touch. Mrs Friend was far too able a woman not to spot her short comings, but too wise to discuss them.

All leave was cancelled over the Dunkirk period, but the expected troubles did not materialise. Romance flourished. Gladys my 'UCH' friend wakened me at midnight to tell me that she had become engaged to her houseman, a Londoner! So, Miss Leslie, she and I went shopping in London. Coupons were of more importance than prices and there was not a lot of choice. Food rationing was biting and restaurants were only allowed to charge 5 shillings for food at any meal. With that in mind we went to a better restaurant than our finances merited. We had not anticipated that the cover charge and other extras would bring the price up to more or less its normal amount!

Gladys had local friends who provided the reception, so hers was very much a hospital wedding. As their contribution some guests had brought bottles which apparently got emptied into an innocuous fruit cup, the staple drink. When we were ready to leave we found a young houseman, a teetotaller, sound asleep in the garden!

Never in all my life had I been able to enjoy work and play as I did that summer of 1941. Gladys left on her marriage, but Haymeads was only a small cog in a vast machine and change ran throughout. At The London Hospital itself, Miss Reynolds retired and Miss Clare Alexander was appointed Matron in her place.

Throughout her forty year 'reign' Miss Lückes had seen Londoners become Matrons of hospitals all over the country, but she herself had been succeeded by Miss Monk, her senior assistant, similarly replaced in her turn by her assistant, Miss Littleboy. In some ways 'The London' seemed to have stood still for twenty years - now the awakening had begun.

I had known Clare for some years. In the second year of her training she had what was known as a 'staff gap' (Staff Nurses' duties in the absence of a Staff Nurse) on night duty in Turner, when I was Staff Nurse in the adjoining Charrington. In theory, each was entirely independent. In practice, a staff nurse was expected to help the holder of a gap as required and in the course of our duties we met in the common lobby. Academic achievement was held in low esteem and I teased Clare about being a 'Prize Pro' (one of the top three in her year's Hospital Final Examinations) 'Prize Pro, Prize Fool' was the taunt! I was however fully aware of her capabilities. Later, when I was a Ward Sister, it was Clare, by then The London's first qualified Sister Tutor, who persuaded me, too, to qualify as a Tutor. By the time I returned she had become Matron of 'Addenbrookes' at Cambridge, where I had visited her from Haymeads.

At the beginning of the war I had told Miss Reynolds that I wanted to join the Navy. It had been a shock to be told that there was a war on and that what I wanted was nothing to do with it. She was, of course, right. Tutors were needed as never before and those who had joined the services were released. It was however another shock when Clare told me that I was to take over as Sister in Charge of the Preliminary Training School.

The London Hospital had been the first hospital in England to introduce a Preliminary Training School. Opened in 1895 at a house in Bow, Miss Lückes considered the six week course would accustom the new probationer to the discipline of hospital life while in a home atmosphere.

By 1923, when I started training, the school had moved to a purpose built school, Tredegar House, in Bow, just two miles from the hospital. It was an intensive course, not so much as a day off for seven weeks, from which we emerged disciplined. The course had changed little in the years. The Sister in Charge taught Nursing subjects in addition to running the school. A Domestic Science teacher, strangely enough attired in Sister's uniform, taught Anatomy and Physiology, Hygiene and Invalid Cookery on which great emphasis was laid.

For two years, in the early 1930s, when I was in charge of the Ante-natal and Gynaecological Out Patient Departments, which did not merit a full time holder, I spent four evenings a week at 'Tredegar' supervising study periods for the half of the students not involved in either Practical Nursing or Bandaging classes. 'The London' made no allowance for such of their trainees as were already qualified in any other branch of nursing e.g. sick children or fevers - all had to go through Tredegar and tormenting me was one of the major relaxations of these groups - one or two, most notably Ella Scott (Dent) ultimately became among my best friends.

From the time of our appointments as Tutors, Miss Harris and I had conducted the 'Tredegar' examinations. After the outbreak of war we continued to do this, first at Hylands and then for the one set housed there at Plaw Hatch.

My set had been the last to be used to make up the numbers for that year's Hospital Classes'. While at Tredegar, we had gone up to 'The London' every Wednesday night for the weekly lecture which was the basis of the year's course. We sat the first hospital examination before we had been in hospital a fortnight. Consequently, our academic careers were undistinguished in the extreme. My last contact with my Tutor, Miss Saunders, had been when I presented my Final State Examination entry form for her signature. State Registration was not even encouraged in the twenties. She told me. 'you deserve to fail and I hope you will'. Much as I resented it, it undoubtedly provided the incentive I needed!

I had never thought of her since, so her letter, congratulating me on my new appointment and outlining the opportunities it provided, took me completely by surprise - it was as apposite as our last exchange had been!

The war and life at Haymeads had widened my horizon - this was different. Laying the foundations of tomorrow's Londoners was a challenge and a responsibility the enormity of which came over me by degrees. In an isolated unit, in war conditions there was the additional responsibility for the students' physical well being - it was a daunting prospect.

CHAPTER FOUR

MERRYMEADE

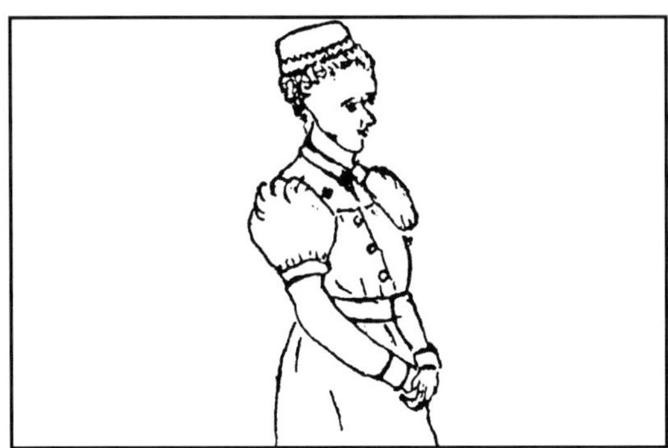

It was autumn when I reached Merrymeade, a large family house on the edge of Brentwood, the property of Mrs Horne Payne. My room was fragrant with late chrysanthemums from the garden which adjoined Brentwood Cricket Ground. It seemed that the Horne Paynes were keen cricketers and had been wont to participate in Cricket Teas! Large country houses, as opposed to Stately Homes, were designed for a family - and the staff who waited on them. They were never intended for mass occupation. At Plaw Hatch the flaw was the water supply. Merrymeade was not on main drainage. I am inclined to think that the latter was the worse.

A massive change over was about to take place. Both Miss Morley, the Sister in charge and Miss Davies, the Domestic Science teacher who had been there for so long, were leaving. The latter was to be replaced by a Dietitian Housekeeper, who would teach Hygiene, Dietetics and Invalid Cookery. As Sister in charge I would teach Anatomy and Physiology as well as Theory and Practice of Nursing. All this was to be phased in and when she arrived in the New Year, I was delighted to hand over the catering to Miss Joan Branson, BSc. Pip, as she came to be known, had trained at King's College of Household and Social Science where I had taken my Tutor Training. Her younger sister had been a Medical Secretary at Haymeads and had married a houseman, so Pip and I had a good deal in common.

The course had been lengthened to eight weeks - every 8th Friday a set left, a new one arrived every 8th Monday. The students were free from 1pm every Saturday until 10pm on Sunday. Miss Muriel Hill, later Principal Tutor, had acted as Assistant for about a year - she was to be replaced by a Junior Sister, based at Merrymeade who would help with practical instruction but was also to be

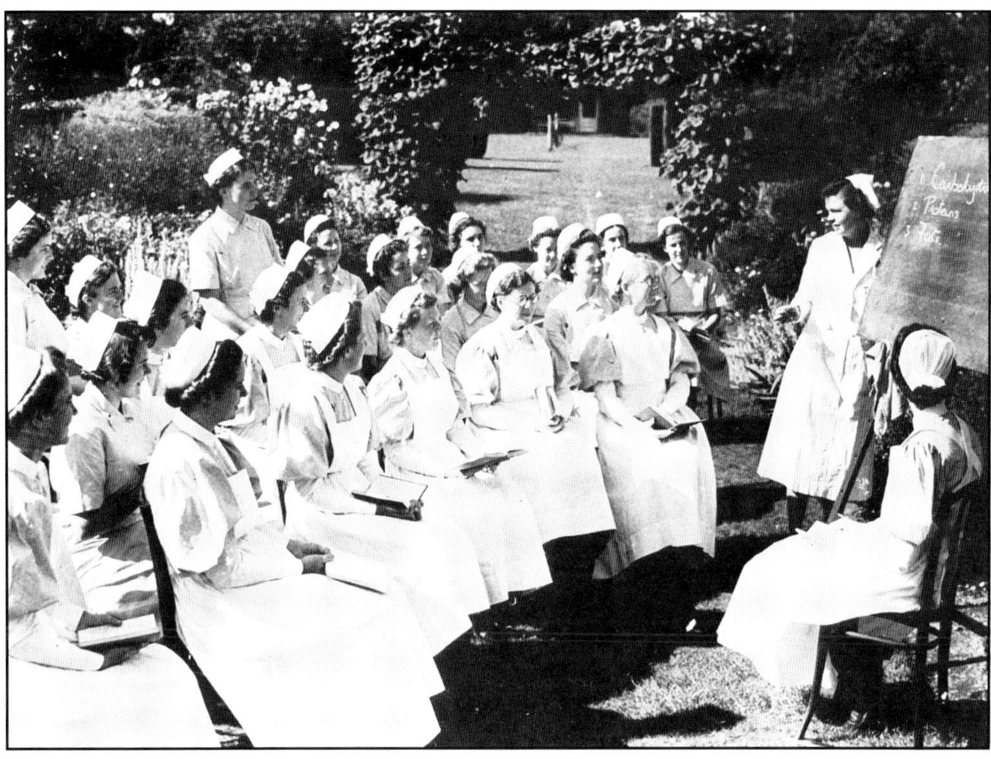

Merrymeade Miss Joan Branson, Bsc. dietitian housekeeper, lectures to the nursing students 1943

the Tutor to the Nurses at Warley a couple of miles away. The only other person involved in the team was Mr Fowler, a member of the Warley staff, who gave every set a course of lectures on gas warfare. I had first attended a gas course' in the summer of 1939. Convinced that such a thing could never happen I had not given it the attention I should and remained confused no matter how often I received the lectures. Mr Fowler also supervised what can best be described as survival technique. All our students slept on the first floor and he insisted that they should be able to get out should both staircases prove impassable. For one room, this involved a canvas shute, demonstration of which was always a source of hilarity.

It was a somewhat spartan life. Until Miss Alexander persuaded Mrs Horne Payne to give us the use of her drawing room, used for storing furniture, both classrooms were situated in the attics and were cold and gloomy. Baths were limited to one a week, to prevent overloading the drainage system rather than on account of shortage of hot water.

It was difficult to introduce much variety into our classes. Pip took every set round the outside of the house studying drain pipes and also to the local sewage works. Rationing restricted the practice of invalid cookery, the results of which were consumed at the next meal. When the Preliminary Training School was first opened, Lord Knutsford, Chairman of the Hospital and an astute business man as well as 'Prince of Beggars', had obtained a London County Council grant for it as an educational establishment. So, once a year we were visited by an Inspector, who would have found it hard to be unduly critical of any evacuated group.

The London Hospital van called once a week and supplied the bulk of our food. A local butcher held our meat ration cards and Merrymeade garden yielded, somewhat grudgingly we felt, a certain amount of fruit and vegetables. As an educational establishment - our students came into the eighteen year old category - we qualified for just one extra - an unlimited supply of sweetened milk cocoa powder. With 7 o'clock breakfast, 'elevenses' were essential. The cocoa was generally popular and infinitely preferable to the alternative - Marmite!

The London Hospital Annexe at Brentwood was about a mile away, but our contact with them was minimal. The medical officer in charge of the health of the nursing staff also covered Merrymeade and all the students' immunisations were given there. In dire emergency we could call on their maintenance staff. I think the only time I ever did so was when the key of one of the lavatories broke in the lock. I had handed coffee and the daily paper through the window, but neither Mrs Horne Payne's gardener nor I could get in through it and to break the door down had seemed unduly drastic.

Mrs Horne Payne and her companion had moved into one of the two staff cottages in the grounds, Smith, her gardener lived in the other. The result was that the School was constantly under surveillance. I did sympathise with her, but the thirty healthy young women, the most that the house could hold, inevitably caused considerable wear and tear. She had not gone to the lengths of Mrs Hanbury, who had had her carpets turned upside down, but there was nothing she missed. In the dining room among the furniture left was a massive dark oak sideboard. The salt and pepper pots were kept in one of its cupboards. Quite soon after my arrival, clearing up after supper one night, one girl had the sideboard cupboard door wide open while she put the salt and pepper pots into it, another with a loaded tray walked straight into the open door, wrenching it off its hinges. It was certainly the most traumatic disaster in the whole of my time there. Open confession was obviously the only step to take. Brandishing my torch I made my way through the black-out to her cottage. I could imagine the commotion there would have been if one of us had done such a thing in my home. My brothers and I always sought to waylay my father on his way in if we had something awful to confess. I wondered if this disaster would have been easier if Mr Horne Payne had been alive. However, Mrs Horne Payne appreciated my gesture and next morning I had to tell the House Governor at The London Hospital of an impending expensive repair. They both said the same thing 'Why do you use those cupboards!'

Merrymeade had however one incomparable asset - the most wonderful housemaid I have ever met. Ellen had been a housemaid at Eton and was used to looking after house masters. Early in the war, I hankered after an enamel dressing table set. Both my sisters had them and it dawned on me that unless I was quick I never should. When next in London I took myself to Mappin & Webbs - they gave The London Hospital staff 10% discount. They had one such set left - the assistant assured me there would be no more. 'Was it', he enquired, 'my husband who had looked at it and said he would get his wife to come and see it!' It was £40 - my annual salary was £160. I bought it, hand mirror, two hair brushes, two clothes brushes and a silver mounted comb. How many English women can have had such an extravagance kept in pristine condition for them all through the war? That, however, was only a minor point. During the bombing no matter how much of the night we had spent up, Ellen would call me at the usual time with not a hair out of place. She took us - the trained staff - at Merrymeade to her heart and waited on us hand and foot. There was no glamour attached to running a Preliminary Training School during a war, but Ellen's service made it much easier.

Pip and I met recently to try to find out why we both look back so happily on our time at Merrymeade. We worked extremely hard, breakfast was at 7 o'clock and either she or I turned out the lights at 10.30 every evening. We had no social life and Pip says she was frightened of coming down the lane leading to the house in the blackout. Domestic help was difficult. If we had no cook, we managed between us, exchanging vital instructions about 1 o'clock dinner as one went into and the other came from the Classroom at noon. The Practical Classroom floor had bare boards, which got filthy. When there was no cleaner, she and I scrubbed half each between sets. My youngest sister, complete with a crawling baby, once filled in as cook for a couple of weeks!

The eighteen year olds that formed the bulk of our intake were marvellous. They just accepted whatever happened and certainly never complained - my admiration for everybody who trained during the war is boundless. The drainage system broke down at intervals. The first time it happened to me, Mrs Horne Payne suggested had somebody tried to flush away a baby! I was outraged, chiefly on behalf of 'my girls' but personally as well. I saw far too much of them to miss such a thing. I can remember standing by the gaping hole - Captain Brierley, the House Governor, somebody from 'The London's' works department, a local dignitary, Smith and me - the whole so closely resembling a burial I thought surely somebody would pray. Fortunately, repairs were always done speedily.

There was an air raid shelter in the basement, which could - just - accommodate the whole household sitting huddled together. Eighteen year olds need their sleep, which left me facing a dilemma every time the siren sounded. The course was an intensive one, there was no time for the students to be dropping off to sleep half way through classes. Had there been room for them to lie down in the shelter I would have marshalled them there every time. One attic window facing towards London was my private look-out post. It was there I decided - rouse the household or not. My abiding horror - unlikely as it was - supposing we had a direct hit, how could I face grieving parents.

'The proper study of mankind is man' dates from the eighteenth Century. Certainly Pip and I found it so, every set was different, all were absorbing. It was Muriel Hill, soon after my arrival, who was convinced that one of the students had previous - undisclosed - nursing experience. She went further and insisted that a close look at her duty shoes confirmed this. Finally I asked the girl, not had she nursing experience, but where. She was so surprised she said, 'Guy's'! Muriel maintained that that girl had found the perfect way of avoiding national service - go through a Preliminary Training School, leave shortly after entering hospital and repeat! Alas! we never knew.

Another time an irate ward Sister rang me up. 'Did we teach the girls nothing at 'Tredegar" - the pre-war name never lapsed. She had found her latest student nurse preparing tea for the patients by mixing dry tea-leaves and milk to a paste at the bottom of the teapot. Onto this she proposed to pour boiling water. The offence was made worse by the fact that the ration of both milk and tea was ridiculously small. The trainees were taught how to make coffee, cocoa and any other substance from which drinks were concocted, but somehow it had always been taken for granted that every eighteen year-old could make tea. I blamed myself, I knew that the girl had lived abroad and had had to be taught the simplest domestic tasks. So, tea making was included from then on.

Busy as we were with preparations, Pip and I always enjoyed the weekend between sets. One sunny Sunday we were having a leisurely tea in the garden, congratulating ourselves on being so well in hand, when we heard a car come up the drive. It stopped at the front door and disgorged two passengers - one of the next day's set, brought by her father, one day early!. Not only was he reluctant to admit that he could be wrong, but his sister, the girl's aunt, was a 'Londoner' about six months my senior! There was nothing for it but to accept the poor girl with a good grace - actually I felt extremely sorry for her and both Pip and I did our best to make her feel welcome. I sent her shopping in Brentwood the next morning and after lunch suggested she should tell the others that she had been the first to arrive - and certainly not for the time being say when. The incident was never referred to again.

A new element of professionalism was emerging. 'The London's training was to be geared to the requirements of the General Nursing Council. The first change was in the students 'Record of Practical Work' - the 'White Book'. This had always been issued when the student had completed six months training and was her responsibility. She must obtain a Sister's signature against every item stating that she had carried out that procedure. Even when I trained several had been virtually obsolete! The new record, the 'Blue Book', based on the official General Nursing Council Schedule, put the onus on the teacher not the taught. Blue Books were among material sent to me before the arrival of each set and it was my responsibility to see that the students left Merrymeade signed up as proficient in such skills as could be taught and practised without patients.

Report forms came next. The authorities in nurse training schools were responsible for giving every student the practical experience demanded by the General Nursing Council. At the same time all wards must be adequately staffed. This juggling act was known as allocation'. Ward Sisters reported briefly to the Sister in charge of allocation every morning. A report on the student's progress in her practical experience was vital; this had always been given verbally, by the Ward Sister to the Sister in charge of allocation, never a wholly satisfactory method. On the form, in addition to the space for the Sister's signature, was a statement to be signed by the student, that she had read the report. Later, in Matron's Office, I learned much of the intricacies involved. At Preliminary Training School level, the report remained confidential and unsigned. Each was filed with the student's papers. Years later, writing references, I always turned back to the first report. It was interesting to read how often they closely resembled later ones.

Clothes rationing in 1941 took the country by surprise and precipitated another change - the amount of material used for uniform must be drastically reduced. Rumour has it that at the turn of the century London Hospital nurses put in a petition - they wanted a more attractive uniform - could they not have the fashionable leg-of-mutton sleeves? The House Committee's decision was that the change could be made but it must be permanent. With the passage of time there was a modest shortening of skirts - eight inches from the floor was the standard when I started training otherwise it remained unchanged. At interview, successful candidates had always been given a parcel containing sufficient material to make four dresses, detailed instructions as to making and a list of other requirements, aprons, sleeves and collars. Caps were provided on arrival.

Miss Alexander tackled this new problem with characteristic thoroughness. Authorities were consulted, sketches submitted and an experienced dressmaker engaged to head a new Uniform Department. All uniform would be made in the hospital. The new dress was a delightful modern - and economical - version of the old. While retaining the original 'puffs' it was complete in itself. Aprons were to be worn only in the wards - a soft turndown collar replaced the stiff one. Each candidate was professionally measured and the uniform really fitted. Miss Pannell came from the Uniform Department to Merrymeade and measured each one. I taught them how to make up and wear their caps - and finally made sure all the new uniform was marked with its owner's name before she left for hospital.

As the war progressed the pressure on 'The London' increased and we too tried to take our share. Miss Alexander supported, encouraged and, one of her most endearing attributes, always gave credit when it was due. When the Chairman, Sir William Goschen, had pneumonia Merrymeade seemed a good place for his convalescence. It was ideal, Ellen was able was able to give him a standard of service which he agreed was rapidly becoming obsolete. I vacated my bedroom, formerly Mr Horne Payne's dressing room, which with a coal fire was all anyone could ask! He was an interesting guest. On one occasion we were discussing changing rates of pay. He said that when first he married he and his wife considered that one could get a really good parlourmaid - for £18 a year!

Under the terms of her appointment, Pip was to be available to lecture to student nurses at 'The London' as required. This happened several times but was never allowed to disrupt the Merymeade routine. I, for one term, taught the Sixth Form Pre-Nursing Course at the local High School. I once went to pick up my bicycle from the school's shed and found there had been a police inspection. The label on mine, 'to the parents of this child', stated that the brakes were in good order but would they please provide an adequate bell! Actually it was Smith, the gardener, who cared for my bike. Every morning I found it clean, the tyres pumped up, and facing the door ready to go!

In spite of rationing and disturbed nights, the health of the Merrymeade students was consistently good. They were vaccinated against small pox before the course started and typhoid was the only one of the immunisations to produce regular casualties. The Practical Nursing Classes were held in the early evening, between five and seven o'clock, and I got to know when to expect disaster - even to planning a class demanding a minimum of standing It was seldom however that ill effects lasted into the next day.

Early one morning, I was awakened by a timid tap on my door. One of the student nurses, a responsible sensible girl, had come to tell me she thought she had mumps! Fortunately the matter was no problem. The girl was an only child, her parents lived relatively near and were happy to look after her. On Sunday afternoon, three weeks later, I had cycled up to Warley a couple of miles away to see some of my friends, when I became conscious of a niggling pain in my jaw. By midnight I was sure - I, too, had mumps! The problem was what to do with me. The medical registrar sent from 'the Annexe' to see me knew no more than I did about mumps, but he had definite views on my disposal. Where did I live and what family would there be at my home? It was illegal to travel by public transport with an infectious disease. Nobody would have petrol to waste on a journey that long and finally, as I had to admit that my youngest sister and her small son were temporarily based at my home, I could not go there anyway. There was nothing for it but the local isolation hospital.

In the second year of my training I had spent six unhappy weeks learning how not to nurse, in a fever hospital, with scarlet fever. I was older now and would have no nonsense! It was bitterly cold - the ambulance men who came to collect me said that the warmest place would be in the front with them so I had a matey journey between the two of them. 'Billericay' was a small isolation hospital with a couple of wards and a row of single cubicles opening onto a veranda. It was very basic. The heating was by open fires - the one in my room was newly lighted. The chilliness of the room was equalled by that of my reception. If I was out for my rights, they were not welcoming. Left to myself I undressed and got into bed. A few minutes later I got up and put on a vest - during the war everybody wore warm vests in winter. Still cold, I added the thick polo-necked jumper I'd arrived in! Finally, a night nurse looked in, bearing a blanket. She said the only other patient admitted that day was a Sergeant Major, also with mumps, and she'd found him in bed with his overcoat on - perhaps I too was cold?

Next morning I was awakened at the crack of dawn by an elderly porter who had come to light my fire and replenish the coal scuttle. Physically I was warm, but the frigid atmosphere remained. It was Sister's day off, it was also the cook's day off, so Matron would not be round as she herself was the relief cook - and a very good one. Next day Sister appeared. She had been a victim of an early bombing and had lost a leg. Finally, she unbent. They had recently had the Theatre Sister from one of the adjacent hospitals as a patient. She had been extremely tiresome and before Sister went for her day off she had told her staff that they were to begin as she meant to go on and to stand no nonsense. I told her my side and from then on all was well. A couple of days later a child with diphtheria was put into the cubicle next to me. What does one do when a child cries in the night? The one night nurse seemed to spend most of her time in the ward block, across the garden. Did I, in the blackout, with no torch and not knowing the way, set out to look for her? Or what? When night nurse finally appeared she wanted to know - how did the child's light come to be on? At least the child had gone to sleep.

The cubicle on my other side was occupied by a patient with meningitis. I was interested to know how cross-infection was avoided. Admittedly no self-respecting germ would leave its warm cubicle for the freezing veranda, but what about crockery and other utensils? Sister assured me that everything used by every patient was kept entirely separate - and washed up individually. Well, but still considered infectious, I carried my tea tray back to the kitchen. My friend the Sergeant Major had taken charge. His jacket off, up to his elbows in hot, soapy water, he seized my crockery and put it in with the rest, mumps, diphtheria, meningitis and who knows what else! I remembered the saying of a wise old physician - God gave us eyes - and lids to close them with!' I never set foot in the kitchen again. Mumps was boring and time wasting and just as I resumed work my assistant developed it! Of all the infectious diseases it must be the most annoying.

I was very sorry, though glad for her, when Pip left to take a post far more worthy of her talents - in Leicester. There, instead of Merymeade's thirty, she catered for 500 patients and 250 staff and battled with the resident medical staff over their ration books and with the cook, who had been there thirty five years. Her replacement, Miss Halley, was young and, at first, a bit lost. About the same time Miss Alexander told me that recruitment was good, the need for nurses great and she was opening a second Preliminary Training School. I was to compile a complete list of the equipment that would be required. Trueloves, about five miles further out was opened in 1944.

Trueloves was much more isolated than Merrymeade. My girls had easy access to both trains and buses; those at Trueloves seemed to be dependent on - and very good at - 'hitching'. I usually cycled there, but on one occasion Annie Harris and I had gone out together and were returning, Annie to 'The London' and me to Merrymeade. The motorist who gave us, both in uniform, a lift volunteered the information that he would be passing 'The London'. To my surprise Annie wouldn't accept and I left her, waiting in Brentwood High Road for the next bus!.

Winter mornings were very dark when 'Summertime' became year long. Now and again the maids overslept and I would be awakened by the sound of the doorbell - the cleaning lady demanding admission. This time, as I opened the door, a man ran down the steps and into an awaiting car which drove off at speed. I looked at my watch - it was 2 o'clock in the morning. Why did I ring up 'the Annexe'? Did I really think the answer lay there or was I seeking comfort? The Night Porter was an old friend of mine - he had been one of the junior Night Porters when I was a junior Night Sister. Anyway, nothing abnormal was going on - certainly they had no link with this. I had not anticipated that my call would feature on Hillman's report to the House Governor. The House Governor's call was unexpected - 'had I notified the police?' Night raids on empty houses were relatively common. The police - as ever - were reassuring 'don't open the door, but ring us'.

Two o'clock next morning the doorbell rang, so I obediently telephoned the police - 'We'll send a man up, but don't open the door'. Next, the back doorbell rang. Stupid as it seems I was terrified!! Surrounded by healthy, active young people, even if they were all asleep, nothing was likely to happen, but the fact remained. However, then the telephone rang, it was the police, the voice said would I open the back door and bring whoever was there to the telephone. My would-be intruder was a Special Constable, told to keep an eye on the house, he was taking the request literally! The following night I was again wakened at 2 o'clock in the morning - by the air-raid siren. I was positively glad - it was reassuring to go back to a familiar situation.

The Physiotherapy School had been completely disrupted by the war, so when a gymnasium at Brentwood Boys School, suitable for practical training, became available, it was decided that the School should be based at Merrymeade, retaining only Trueloves as a Preliminary Training School.

The set that left just before Christmas in 1944, was Merymeade's last and I reopened it in the New Year to Physiotherapy Students. They were to live and have their lectures at Merrymeade, Brentwood School was within easy walking distance for practical work, as was the Annexe. Their Tutors, Miss Dena Gardiner and Miss Joan Barker were also resident and I became a sort of Home Sister. An hour's housework every morning had always been part of the student nurses' practical experience. There was no domestic staff to cover this, so the practice continued. My personal conviction was that it was good for Physiotherapy Students to know how to make a bed properly and a basic knowledge of cleaning can never come amiss. I found Physiotherapy Students much like Student Nurses, my most vivid memory is of identical twins who delighted in confusing us - I had spent three happy years at Merrymeade, but the war in Europe was over and so too was my work there. Change was in the air and I looked forward to taking part in the development of post war nurse training.

CHAPTER FIVE

WARTIME AT 'THE LONDON'

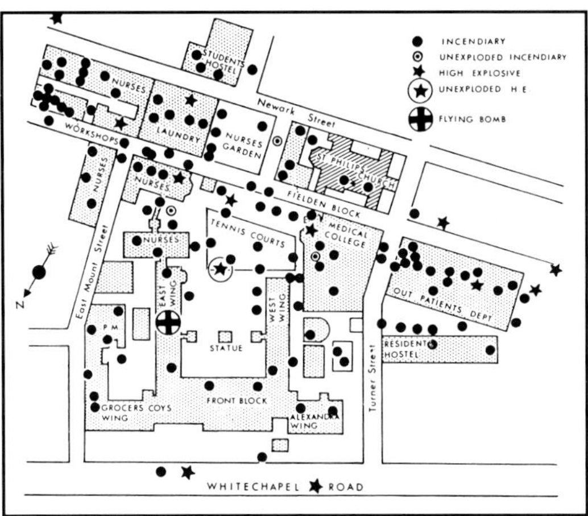

Bombs on the Hospital World War II

Even in 1939 the priorities of nurse training were changing. From being entirely the province of the Ward Sister, some practical nursing was to be taught in the Classroom. 'The London's' only Practical Classroom, situated over the laundry, was excellently equipped - for the teaching of Invalid Cookery. A row of sinks and another of gas cookers, a fixed demonstration area with gas hot plate and tiered seating formed an unlikely background for bedsteads, trolleys and bulky equipment. Preparing for a practical nursing examination I had remarked to Annie Harris that it needed a bomb on it.

On September 8th 1940 I came from Bishops Stortford to help with the following week's nurses' examinations. As we reached Liverpool Street the air-raid sirens sounded. At Aldgate everybody was turned off the District Line train and directed to the nearest shelter. This seemed to be no place for me and the Warden in charge agreed I could go on to 'The London'. A few yards down the road I was accosted by a plain clothes policeman, who took my case and said he would walk me to 'the Hospital'. Having said, "When I say duck, duck," he proceeded to tell me how he had come to join the police - until he did say, "Duck". We both ducked and our backs were sprinkled with bits of flying glass. Dusting me down he continued calmly with the half finished sentence and in due course we parted at the front gate - but ever after whenever I heard the siren I was grateful to him.

That was right at the beginning of the Blitz - the night a bomb fell through the Classroom and exploded in the Laundry. With several other people I spent the rest of the night in the entrance hall of the Old Home. Early the next morning Annie Harris found me there and stated baldly, 'You've had your wish'. Looking at the damage, it seemed as if with a bit of tidying the examination could have proceeded on the edges surrounding the jagged hole. However, by midday Annie and I were at the Chase Farm Unit at Enfield preparing for the examination, only slightly delayed, to be held there.

Mrs Doreen Cook (nee Lilley) 1941 - 1945 writes in detail of the war years:-

'By 1944 the East end of London had endured the ravages of the Blitz in 1940/41 and the daylight bombing raids of 1942/43. The London Hospital had taken in the casualties; the Duty medical teams dealt with the wounded - minor cuts and bruises to be dressed and the patients sent home; the more serious to be X-rayed and admitted for possible surgery. The operating theatres were alerted and emergency contingency plans put into action.

Meanwhile the Surgical Consultants completed their normal operation lists and the routine work in the theatres continued to be done. Miss Ida Latham, the Sister-in-Charge of the Operating Theatres, presided over this busy - sometimes hectic - scene with efficiency and humour and her staff responded in like manner!

D-Day, June 6th came and went, but now The London was to face a more formidable and terrifying ordeal - pilotless missiles - the V1's or 'flying bombs' and V2's or 'rockets'. From 12th June 1944 to the end of March 1945, 2420 flying bombs fell on London - 30 in Stepney, 9 in Bethnal Green and 17 in the City of London, while 570 V2 rockets reached the London area. The devastation was enormous, the casualty lists high and death tolls rising. 'The London' had its share of the deeply shocked and wounded cases admitted to the Receiving Room and First Aid Post for treatment and possible surgery. The Air Raid Sirens gave some warning of the approach of a 'doodle bug' - at 1.30am on August 3rd, one fell on the hospital killing two patients in Royal Ward - but the V2 was a sudden violent explosion and the sound of falling masonry.'

Mrs Ella Scott (nee Dent) was the Dietitian and, like everybody else the night that Royal was hit, was up. She and Mr Bowler, the Catering Officer, decided special measures were called for - at 3.30am they embarked on preparing a REAL breakfast. She writes:-

'The patients had boiled eggs - this relieved the junior nurses from their kitchen duties to help in their wards. For the staff it was bacon and egg, but, alas! no toast. The cooking was done by me, a junior Sister and two Dining Room Supervisors. It was an unheard of luxury in wartime and did a tremendous amount to boost the morale of everybody. It was a worthwhile effort - when the staff arrived their faces were a joy to see - amazement and appreciation!'

Mrs Cook, who began her year as a Staff Nurse in the Operating Theatres in the spring of 1945, describes a V2 Rocket Incident:-

'In March there were a number of V2 rocket explosions in the vicinity of the hospital and we were on constant alert to deal with the casualties. One Friday afternoon we were just finishing the last surgical list of the week when there was a violent explosion; the lights dimmed and the windows shook but, luckily, did not shatter. The Assistant Surgeon finished the abdominal stitching, applied the dressing; the anaesthetist pronounced himself satisfied with the patient's condition; I was clearing my trolley, stacking the instruments into the tray for subsequent cleaning and resterilising. The patient was lifted on to the theatre trolley to be taken to the ward.

Sister came into the theatre to announce that casualties were being admitted to the wards and we must be ready for the Surgical staff to operate as soon as possible. All the staff hurried to clear up the two theatres that had been used for the afternoon lists; the floors and operating tables to be swabbed with carbolic; the Boyles apparatus to be checked and prepared for the first casualty. Emergency sets of instruments were boiled in the steriliser (at that time only orthopaedic instruments for Sir Reginald Watson-Jones were autoclaved! We also boiled up syringes for re-use - they were stored in trays of spirit).

Sister, two staff nurses (including myself) and four probationers remained on duty. In turn, we were sent off for an early supper. Miss Uren, the Catering Officer, was always ready with emergency meals. Night staff nurse and two probationers came on early; the Duty Registrar (Mr Tanner) with the Duty Anaesthetist and housemen came along the theatre corridor and by 7.30pm we were ready for the first patient.

We divided into teams. Mr Tanner dealt with the most serious injuries mainly caused by flying glass which pitted the skin and was often deeply embedded into the flesh. Most of the patients had bled profusely, were in deep shock and were on blood transfusions. An Orthopaedic Registrar dealt with fractured limbs and surface injuries in the second theatre. The duty housemen were scrubbed up to assist.

We finished at about 3.30am. Thirteen patients had been operated upon. The teams had worked well together, snatching meals or cups of tea when they could, between operations. Sister's calm efficiency had been very evident. I had scrubbed up for some of the operations and even helped Mr Tanner to stitch up some of the wounds - a job usually done by a student! But this night they had been occupied in the First Aid Post or helping to ferry the casualties to and from the theatres! After the last patient had been returned to the ward, we nurses cleared the theatres, tied up the dirty linen, washed and cleaned the instruments; leaving one theatre ready for the next emergency. We were very tired but Sister was pleased and at 5am we went off for tea and bed.

On March 26th and 27th two more V2's exploded near the hospital and more casualties were admitted.

On March 29th, the last V1 fell near Orpington in Kent. The missile raids were over. The end of the war was in sight'.

Daphne Elliott - Crossman Night Probationer - remembers, 'The night a land mine fell on Whitechapel Underground Station' (a night between April 3rd and May 10th 1944).
She writes:-

'Staff Nurse Jean Aitken and I were on night duty in Crossman Ward situated on the ground floor of the hospital and facing Whitechapel Road. As was customary during this period we began work in an empty ward preparing for the nightly reception of casualties. Usually by about midnight all beds would be full of patients injured in the night's air raids. In the morning these were transferred to other wards or one of the Sector hospitals. This was the time when incendiary bombs were being dropped. They caused enormous fires and terrible casualties many of whom suffered from severe burns. Often people were trapped and burned in surface air raid shelters as well as in other buildings. Facial burns were common. Face masks covered the dressings and it needed great patience and compassion to guide people who had come to identify their relatives and friends and were bewildered by the identical masked faces in every bed. At this time too, limbs with first and some second degree burns were often encased in "Bunyan's Bags" i.e. - plastic sleeves with nozzles firmly secured round limbs. They were filled with a warm solution of Milton in which the burnt part could literally float. Many such burns healed cleanly and without scarring.

Sometime after midnight, the ward was full after the regular evening bombardment, we heard an unusually loud bang and bumping which sounded as though the hospital had received a direct hit above us. Staff Nurse Aitken and I looked helplessly at each other and thought that our end had come. Wearing our tin hats and carrying lamps we stood hand in hand in the middle of the ward and waited in trepidation. It turned out to be a mine which landed on Whitechapel Underground Station on the other side of the road. The blast blew in all the blackout and the subsequent fire made the ward as light as day. Recovering from the shock we looked round the ward to find that all the patients who could move at all had dived instinctively under their beds!
The ward floor was awash with Milton and intravenous solutions and it took us the rest of the night, with the help of porters and students to put the patients safely back to bed and restore order.

Miss Elliott was later a Theatre Staff Nurse and has described the Bethnal Green Flying Bomb. One of the first of the flying bombs to hit the London area it fell on Bethnal Green destroying a railway bridge and killing six people.

'The night of June 13th was the only occasion during the whole war when I experienced a momentary terrible fear and panic. We were completing a list in the Private Wards theatre when we heard a plane flying low over the hospital: the engine cut out and seconds later there was a loud crash. Moments later the telephone rang and we were told a plane had come down near the hospital and to prepare the theatre and ourselves for casualties. We did this as quickly as possible and waited and waited. Eventually the telephone rang again and we were told there were no casualties and there was no pilot in the plane. It was our first experience of a flying bomb and I think it was the shock and uncanny realisation that a missile resembling a plane could land anywhere without any homing control which gave the awful feeling that the bottom had dropped out of the world. It was not long of course, before we used to go home in a train, look at a flying bomb out of the window and hope that when the engine cut out it would fall away from the train and not towards it'.

At the height of the flying bomb period Miss Alexander called a meeting of the Sisters involved in teaching at all the Sector hospitals. We met in the old Fourth Floor Classroom where original bomb-damage had been repaired. Half way through we heard an approaching missile - its engines cut out - Miss Alexander said, 'We'll stop for a minute'. Probably all of us had much the same thought - why hold a meeting on a top floor - and then relief -.it fell nowhere near.

My only encounter with a V2 was a miss. Merrymeade was being used for physiotherapy students and I cycled over to Trueloves four evenings a week to help with the teaching of practical nursing. About half way there one night I heard the thud of a rocket behind me - some way off but near enough to raise every hair of my head. Two hours later, cycling back I was stopped by a crater near enough to the road to make it temporarily impassable. Two minutes later on my outward journey and I could have vanished without trace!

The maternity wards were closed at the beginning of the war, opening later with an additional 75 beds in two units, one at Hitchin, the other at Woolmer Park, a large country house situated between Hatfield and Hertford. It was a 'hunting lodge' belonging to the Earl of Strathmore, father of Queen Elizabeth, now the Queen Mother.

F. Elizabeth Williams, a pupil midwife in 1944 describes: 'A long drive with very tall trees topped with mistletoe. It was a place of pretty little dells where woodland flowers grew in profusion, plus tiny streams and heathers. It was a place of natural beauty. My 'town heart' was completely overcome. Miss Ireland was the Sister in charge. The large panelled hall and staircase were very much of the stately house type. On a table in the hall was a book which Miss Ireland insisted must be read.

It was more or less a book of guidance as to what to do - and not do. The contents I cannot remember - the statement on the first page I do - it read: 'This is not Liberty Hall'. It spoke volumes.

I have no recollection of the rooms converted to wards or the labour ward, or where we dined and slept, apart from the one where we slept when on night duty. This was known as The Belfry and for a good reason - the bats also slept there. Seeing the bats hanging from the ceiling was somewhat daunting but presumably they were in residence before the Londoners arrival and were part of life in the country. The other notable room was 'the toilet' (not anymore 'The cottage' - The London's time honoured euphemism). It was a long narrow panelled room with two or three internal stairs, the toilet proper, boxed in with beautiful wood, in the centre of the topmost one. The toilet pan was decorated with a most exquisite floral design. There was no chain to pull or lever to press, encased at the right side was a brass handle, which one pulled up.

One of our midwives had achieved an ambition whilst at Woolmer Park - she became a campanologist, ringing the bells at the Parish Church of Hertingfordbury! Our off duty time was mostly spent on our cycles, visiting the nearby lovely villages, especially Essenden where there was a post office. Buses would take us to Hertford but returning in time for duty was a problem. We were obliged to travel to The London Hospital for lectures. This meant a very early start. The two night nurses changed into mufti and joined the day staff for breakfast. The first bus of the day from Hertford to Hatfield must be caught at the end of the Drive by the House gates. We ran down, eating our breakfast toast and looking through the trees for the coming bus. This took us to Hatfield Station to catch the workman's train to Bethnal Green. I remember the mad dash to Mary Northcliffe to be on time for the first of two lectures. Mr Brews was one of the Chiefs. Efforts to keep awake after a night on duty and the journey meant disaster as far as note taking was concerned. On arrival 'home' we joined the rest of the staff for lunch and, for those on night duty, to bed.

The Practical Exams for Part I took place in October at Brocket Hall, near Welwyn, an Emergency Maternity Hospital belonging to another of the teaching hospitals. Miss Margaret Walker, our tutor, teaching on the 'rickety pelvis' advised me to 'swot up' rickets as Professor Brown, most probably the examiner, always asked about it. The Sister-in-charge recognised 'The London' uniform. She too hoped I knew all about rickets as I should be asked by Professor Brown! When I had examined the patient, the great man posed the inevitable question, but instead of giving a sensible and knowledgeable answer, I said, 'I have never seen a case of rickets, Sir.' He replied, 'Rubbish girl, go up to Glasgow, you can push a wheelbarrow between their legs!!'

The exam results came out in November. I still cherish the reply from Miss Greaves, the Sister in Charge at Brockett Hall, to whom I had written to tell the good news. She hoped I would go on to Part II. I had sent a telegram to Miss Elizabeth Major at 'The London' - I cherish her reply, too, saying I must go on to Part II. Woolmer Park was a happy place.

Dame Phyllis Friend was also a pupil midwife at 'Woolmer'. She recalls that the Night Sister always presented her report to the day staff, not when they came on duty, but as they ate breakfast, no lurid details being omitted!

District midwifery continued throughout the war. With Miss Alma Dear in charge, the midwives replaced their green bonnets with tin hats and carried on as usual. **Jessie Edwards**, (Mrs Frost) was one of them. In 'A Day with Pam the Midwife' she describes a typical day.

'Life was very hectic what with the activities of war, sirens screaming and bombs falling. As a midwife practising in the East End of London it was no easy task coping with war time atrocities. That day she had joined the other four midwives for breakfast. They covered a one mile radius from the hospital. The first call came in at half-past-eight, it was Pam's turn and picking up her bag she hurried to the front hall of the hospital. She recognised the man anxiously awaiting as Mr Hall. They walked side by side, he made no effort to carry her bag. Glancing at him, he would be approaching forty, he was dirty, unshaven and shabbily dressed. He did not speak and she had to run to keep up with him. He lived in a tenement building. 'On the third floor' he gruffly told her.

Many East Enders were evacuated at the beginning of the war, but many stayed, no bombs would move them. There were no lifts in the building and the stairs were steep. On reaching the third floor Mr Hall opened one of the three doors that were spaced on the landing. Pam was well aware of what she would find, two rooms littered with dirty clothing, make-shift furniture and a table which was covered with the remains of a meal.

In the corner of one room lay Mrs Hall on a very badly broken bed, certainly no room for two people. Hearing a small whimper she looked round and under the table she saw a small puppy! Mr Hall found his voice and said 'Here's the nurse, Nell'. Nell didn't answer and it was obvious that she was well advanced in labour. Pam made a space on the table and covering it with newspaper she put down her bag. The door banged, she found Mr Hall had gone.

This was Nell's third confinement, her other two children (girls) were being cared for by the Council until this little one was born. Pam was well acquainted with Nell's past confinements which had been normal deliveries. In view of the appalling conditions everything had been done to persuade her to go to hospital, but she flatly refused. Fortunately there was the usual morning lull in air activity but it wouldn't last. Pam thought of the Tube Dwellers and of those who had lost everything, but the need to survive was strong and all the time there was a glimmer of hope that all would be well.

Nell hadn't attended the ante-natal clinic very often, but Pam hoped the labour would be normal, help was not far away, there was always a doctor on call. Taking off her coat to put on the white gown, she took the kettle to fill it from the tap which was on the landing above. This was the only one which served the three flats. Putting the kettle on the stove, she wished to give Nell a wash, there was no gas, Pam looked hopefully at Nell but knew the answer, luckily she found a shilling in her purse. She helped Nell to wash and she looked reasonably clean in her ragged night-dress. She was making good progress but as Nell's husband had gone Pam thought it would be nice to have someone to call on if help were needed. She knocked on one of the other doors. A middle-aged woman poked her head out, her hair was in curlers and a cigarette was dangling from the corner of her mouth. She stared at Pam, 'Oh hello nurse she's started then?' 'Yes' said Pam, 'her husband has gone out. I was wondering if I need help may I call you?' She laughed, 'I've had nine, you can count on me'.

There was nothing prepared for the baby and looking at the chest of drawers she decided the lower drawer would make a bassinet. She pulled it out. Nell gave a shout, but too late, the chest fell over. Nell thought it very funny. Pam wasn't hurt, but apparently the front leg was broken. The door opened and Nell's husband came in, he said 'I've brought you some fish and chips'. Nell didn't want them, though he urged her to eat to keep her strength up and put the parcel on the table.

The delivery was normal, in fact Pam was very proud of the way Nell coped. The baby was a little girl (Nell wasn't pleased she wanted a boy) she was perfect, did the fish and chips help to build such a lovely little body? Filling the kettle Pam found more money was needed for the meter. What a cruel world it is she thought as she made a cup of tea. Taking off her gown, putting on her coat, picking up her bag, she told Nell she would call back in about four hours. On her return she took clothes for Nell and the baby, both were well. Nell was encouraged to have a check-up after having had daily visits for two weeks but she probably wouldn't bother.'

In the course of the war, all sorts of odd situations arose. This one was relayed to me in instalments - by telephone. The wife of one of my Kent cousins was having a second baby. It cannot have been straight forward, as she was to be admitted to hospital for the birth. The sector hospital concerned was based in a mental hospital. When my cousin arrived to visit he found his wife in a highly agitated state. Her single room was nothing other than a padded cell!

Much to his surprise the midwife in charge inquired if he was related to me. On being told he was, she said, her advice to him was to take his wife elsewhere. That was not easy, but a Nursing Home in Bromley took her. No sooner had the baby been born than the Home was bombed and finally mother and baby reached East Grinstead's only Nursing Home. Next our General Practitioner called on my mother and told her that he was, "not happy about the baby!"

Norah, the elder of my two young sisters, was temporarily at home with her small son. She was developing into a very capable young woman and she had one other great advantage. The London Hospital Private Staff Nurses were first rate midwives, 'Monthly Nurses' was the term for them. They prided themselves that they left young mothers well able to cope and Norah had had one of the best. She had been left with a thriving, contented baby and felt nobody could teach her anything about infant care. Naturally she went and looked at the baby and together with my mother decided they could do better than any Nursing Home - so Norah brought mother and baby home in a taxi. The first thing they discovered was that the Home's idea of changing a baby was to apply another layer - there were five when they first investigated, certainly my family's optimism was justified. In their care, this one too became another thriving contented baby.

My mother hated long distance telephone calls, so I knew something must be wrong when she rang me up. My youngest sister was somewhere in the Montrose area with a baby of about fifteen months old. Her husband had just been posted abroad - and she was in the throes of a miscarriage. Mother demanded that I went and sorted it out and perhaps brought Richard back with me. Miss Alexander was always sympathetic over such problems, her own brother had been killed in action and her sister and mine had met in the maternity wards. She readily gave permission for me to add an extra day on to my weekend and I set out. Cook cut some sandwiches, Ellen said I must take a rug. Pip, whose young sister's life ran a similar course, was glad it was not her! Overnight travel in blacked out trains was not much fun. At some point in the small hours we had to change trains and a serviceman I had met on the way took me with him into the warmth of the refreshment bar provided for the forces - nobody queried that I was not in uniform.

I finally reached Montrose about midday, I found Florence was no longer at the address I had been given. The Minister of the local Church and his wife had taken her and Richard into their own home. Both were perfectly happy. - mine was a completely unnecessary journey. Admittedly their views on feeding a child did not correspond with mine, but love was of far more importance than calories. We all had every reason to be most grateful to them. I had additional cause - the thought of an overnight journey with a child who did not know me had filled me with horror. As it was all I had to do was to embark on the long journey back.

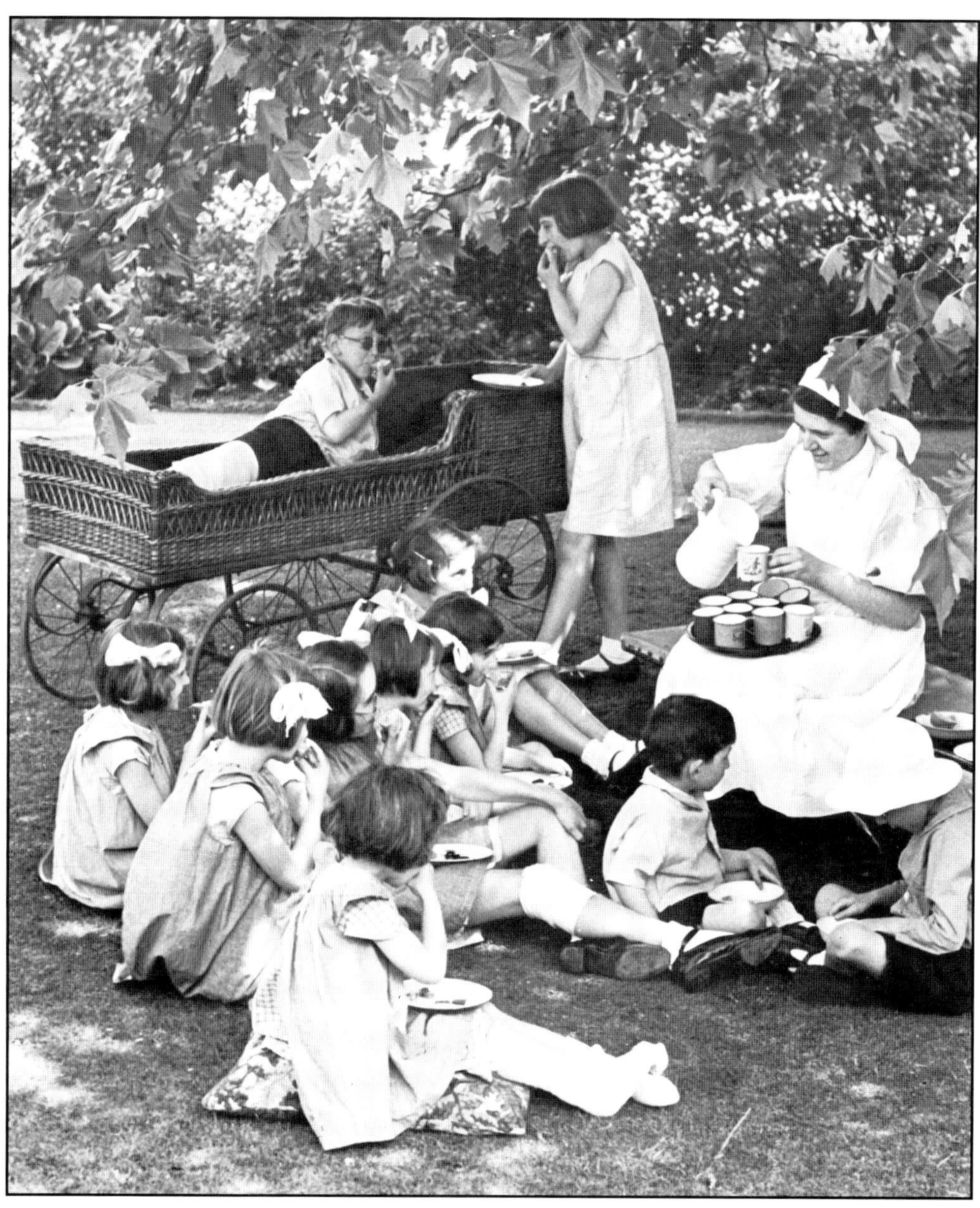

Convalescent children at the Catherine Gladstone House, Mitcham, handed over to the Govenors in memory of the work done at 'The London' by Mrs Gladstone, wife of the Prime Minister during the Cholera Epidemic of 1866.

CHAPTER SIX

BACK AT 'THE LONDON'

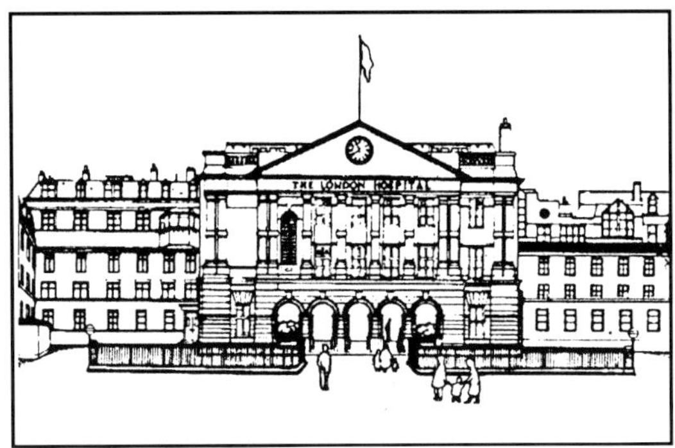

V.E. night (Victory in Europe) was May 9th 1945, shortly before I returned to The London. The only place to be was at the gates of Buckingham Palace, so I travelled up from Brentwood and with thousands of others cheered the King, the Queen and Princess Elizabeth in her khaki uniform. No longer could I, taking Prayers at Merrymeade every morning, intersperse The London Hospital's own prayer with pleas for the men risking their lives to bring us food.

I have vivid recollections of November 11th 1918 - Armistice Day. England was in the throes of an influenza epidemic - in a vain attempt to protect the boarders from infection the day girls were excluded from school. My sisters and I were in the garden at 11 o' clock when the fire hooter went! East Grinstead had a fire engine, but the horses used to draw it were employed on normal council business. So - the fire hooter was the signal for the man on the dust cart or other routine chore to return to base. Eleven o' clock on Armistice Day must have been the only time the hooter was ever put to any other use.

In 1914 England's women had been campaigning for the vote, but abandoning this they worked magnificently all through the war. It was a dreary war - food was rationed, coal was rationed, and every day more men were killed in action, reported missing or wounded, probably for life. My nineteen year old brother, piloting a Bristol Fighter, had been reported missing two months previously. My father's youngest brother, drafted into the Artillery had his jaw blown off before he ever reached his gun position - never again could he eat solid food.

In 1919 The Government of the day generously rewarded England's women by giving them the vote - at the age of thirty! My mother's youngest sister's husband died of cancer in his thirties just before the war. She had no money and no training, but throughout the war she worked happily at the War Office, became engaged to a distant Australian cousin fighting in France and her future seemed assured. As demobilisation got under way, she with all the other women who had kept men's jobs open was dismissed - and the Australian cousin was drowned in a boating accident. Poor Aunt Maude - and there were thousands like her - at forty, the daughter at home entirely dependent on her family.

My brothers, at school in London in the first war, had come home with tales of the Zeppelin raids, a very minor occurrence, but the second was a people's war. There was mass evacuation, wide spread bombing, civilian as well as service casualties. One of my friends had four children, three sons, one in each of the services, but it was their daughter in the Land Army, about whom they had never felt any anxiety, who was killed.

It was not only Nurses and Nursing that the war had changed - women were awakening. I was to a certain extent prepared for change; for the past five years we had all mixed with 'outsiders' in assorted Sector Hospitals. Marriage was no longer taboo! The vast majority of nurses were still unmarried but the subterfuge of the twenties, when a wedding ring could only be worn dangling on a ribbon next to the skin had gone. As a Staff Nurse on night duty, returning to report to the Ward Sister at a quarter to nine in the morning, I knew that one of my fellow Staff Nurses was doing just that. She also walked into the ward with her corridor cape hanging neatly from her folded arms - obscuring the bulge below her apron belt. Birth control was another factor in the changing position of all women, not just nurses. I cannot remember when I first heard:

'Arabella full of 'opes
Bought a book of Marie Stopes
Judging by her sad condition
Fear she bought the wrong edition'.

The first Birth Control clinic was opened in 1920 and the Family Planning Association began in 1930. It would have been in the thirties that a woman in the Ante-natal department told me bitterly, 'to think that I paid 3/6 for a box of them things'. Her husband's weekly wage would have been about a pound.

The move towards professionalism noted at Merrymeade was continuing. Miss Alexander was insistent that only a Tutor should be in charge of the allocation of nurses. Miss Ceris Jones, a Nightingale (St. Thomas's Hospital) was already doing this. Ceris like Miss Alexander - and myself - had taken her Tutor training at King's College. She had worked briefly at Warley Woods and the Brentwood Annexe before joining the Matron's Office team. Miss Alexander had also appointed several Sisters who had been on her staff at Addenbrookes and there was a sprinkling of Australians and New Zealanders who had stayed on in England after serving in the Armed Forces. It was inevitable the 'The London's' 'inbred' only system had ended.

I had been allotted a pleasant bed sitting room overlooking the garden. Domestic service had deteriorated as much in hospital as in private houses, but there was thankfulness everywhere just that the war was over.

My first morning I reported in Matron's Office. The senior night Sister had eloped! London Hospital Sisters didn't do such things, but what could be a more suitable place in which to put an unoccupied experienced Sister! I had been away from 'The London' for nearly six years, even worse, for three and a half years I had not so much as seen a patient. Antibiotics were perhaps the greatest innovation of that time and there was early ambulation. Bed had become something to keep the patients out of, instead of a nurse's worst misdemeanour being to let a bedfast patient put a foot out of his bed.
I spent the morning in a surgical ward, was initiated into the new and vitally important rules for giving drugs and generally brought up to date. The rest of the day was mine - pre-war London Hospital Sisters were avid theatre-goers, and I had not been to a London theatre since 1940. Rather than get frustrated attempting to sleep I took myself up West to a matinee and in due course presented myself with the other Night Sisters in Matron's Office.

The day report we were given contained only one noteworthy incident in my side of the hospital - a very sick small child admitted to one of the children's wards. I took myself there. I might be three and a half years out of practice but I could recognise a dying child when I saw one. He was the son of 'Londoners' whom I knew, there was a young baby at home so his mother could not leave but his father came. My sister had recently lost a baby, also I was out of practice at the professional avoidance of involvement. As the sun rose over the dome of St Pauls the poor little scrap died and his father and I wept together on David Hughes balcony.

The Night Sisters last job was to mark the day nurses into breakfast. Each student nurse gave her name which was ticked off in a massive register. They were practically all my girls who had been through Merrymeade. Seeing me, they beamed and said, "Good morning Sister " - they knew I knew them, so I did, but could I put names to them? All I could do was to put ticks into the register and hope that everyone was there.

Strangely, after that baptism, I enjoyed my fortnight's night duty and it worked wonders in getting me back to hospital routine.

My next move was to Fielden House, 'The Block' adjoining St Philips Church on the far side of Stepney Way. Built as an Isolation Block it had been converted into Private wards in the course of the thirties. My destination was the fourth floor, named St Anthony, this was designed for the overnight admission of patients being treated for syphilis. The rooms were tiled - the walls were washed after every admission. In the '20's a medical Ward Sister, Miss Rose Simmonds had been sent to the United States of America to study dietetics, and on her return St Anthony became the Dietetic Department. I had worked there briefly. One of its features was that all patients' food - they were all on 'Special Diets' - was cooked in the ward kitchen. The Preliminary Training School course of invalid cookery did not really fit the average probationer to produce a 'cut off the joint and two veges' for eighteen or so patients, but we did extremely well. As cooks we, the probationers, considered ourselves entitled to any food that was left over. This applied particularly to the evenings, if we could scrounge a hasty snack between eight and nine o'clock we could get ourselves marked in for nine-thirty supper in the dining room, walk straight through and get ahead in the subsequent queue for baths. One evening Sister caught me consuming cheese and biscuits, she said that she didn't mind us eating if we were hungry, but surely I was spoiling my supper. She had no idea that it was my supper.

During the war 'The Block' had been used to accommodate consultants on call and it was now being reopened for Private Patients. The fourth floor ultimately became the Nurses Sick Room but I was to re-open it as Private Wards. The third floor was already operational. Miss Margaret Anthony, the Sister there, gave me a great deal of help. One of the pearls of wisdom she passed on was that the patients beds must be stripped, and linen and towels removed before they went home, otherwise they took them with them. All household linens were rationed so presumably it was understandable, but it was something of a shock to me.

I had brought my bicycle to London with me. The previous weekend I had cycled to London Bridge Station and left it propped against some railings. When I returned from East Grinstead two days later, the bicycle was there ready for me to ride back to Whitechapel. It was difficult to equate such honesty with sheet stealing.

Nursing in the Private Wards was a new experience. All my hospital experience was of The London's fourteen bed sub wards. The patients could all be seen by the staff - equally the patients could see their nurses and would know how busy they were and when was a good moment to seek attention. In addition, the life of the ward and the other patients were a source of interest. I had experience of Private Nursing, where the patient has his nurse's undivided attention. The Private patient in his single room has inestimable advantages, but is in some ways worse off than either. Alone, by himself, he has nothing to occupy his mind but his ills and, rightly, expects immediate attention when he rings his bell. Above all he loses out on the camaraderie that one finds in a ward. For the nurse, she has to remember that for each Private patient he himself is all that matters. One day we had had an exceptionally busy evening. It was about 10 o'clock when I went into one room to say 'goodnight' to its occupant. She was pleased to see me, 'I've hardly seen you all day dear - sit down and talk to me'. She was, of course, within her rights. My Ward Sister's soul warred with my tutorial one! Before the war, nurses' lectures were given at 8 o'clock in the evening. Now all my nurses seemed to be due in the classroom for a lecture at 9 o'clock in the morning. My Ward Sister's side thought it outrageous that they then did not reappear until nearly 11 o'clock, though my tutorial side tried to accept it.

Domestic help, too, was scarce. At Merrymeade, the students washed up after meals, everything else Ellen did. I found that every patient expected that his friends should be given tea, forty to fifty cups and saucers would accumulate in the kitchen, with no ward maid until 5 o'clock. The wife of one of my patients wanted to talk to me - she was told I was in the kitchen.
She was amazed and said to me, 'my dear, you shouldn't be doing that' as she picked up the tea towel and wiped up as she talked! She dropped in every afternoon of her husband's stay - it hardly seemed right that they should pay heavily and help wash up.

One of my patients was a retired naval man. I had explained to my nurses that his language, geared to the quarter deck, meant nothing and should certainly never be reciprocated. 'Damn and blast you woman', he said to me on one occasion. Concentrating on the stitches I was removing, my reply was pure reflex action, I am not given to swearing, and 'Blast your eyeballs sir', slipped out just as, 'only two more stitches' might have done. If he was startled I was appalled, swearing at patients was an unforgivable sin.
Had he picked up the telephone and repeated to the House Governor what I had said it would have been the end of me. Strangely enough he never swore at me again.

From the private wards I went on holiday. The war was over! Food was rationed - clothing was rationed, but England's beaches were accessible again. My youngest sister's husband was still abroad. She and a friend each with one child were sharing a bungalow at Lancing and I joined them. Both the boys were at the latest stages of whooping cough, no longer infectious but sounding horrific. It was bliss to sit on the beach in the sunshine even though Lancing is not among the more glamorous of the Sussex beaches. There were few visitors. Both the girls were careful to keep away from spots where children were already playing, they had no control over those who came later. Sooner or later, either Richard or Timothy would cough, any mother within ear-shot promptly gathered up her offspring and fled, with baleful looks in our direction.

Back at 'The London', I was told to go to the Linen Room. This was another department that had probably originally been put in charge of a Sister for want of any suitably qualified professional. As the term suggests the Linen Room controlled the linen supply for the whole of the hospital. I was not there long enough to discover whether or not it was a good system financially, otherwise it worked well. Each ward and department had its own linen supply, clearly marked. Every ward or departmental Sister was responsible for her own supply. It was understood that linen in need of, or beyond, repair was put aside. Generally speaking it would have been Sister or her Staff Nurse, who put away the linen returned daily from the Laundry, but nobody, probationer or trained, would put torn linen on a bed. Once a week, such linen was taken to the Linen Room for repair, or to be condemned. Once a year, there was a linen inventory. Conducted by two Assistant Matrons in a mammoth operation every single piece of linen was counted.

Immediately post-war a new system was in the process of introduction. Linen no longer belonged to individual wards or departments. Sisters were not responsible, they merely ordered the linen they needed daily from the Central Supply department. Nurses' hours of duty were shorter, nurses' time was too valuable to be wasted on non-nursing duties. The turnover of patients was more rapid, thus increasing the pressure on linen supplies. A Central Supply must be more economical and effective, but last time I was admitted to hospital I fought with the solid wedge that formed my pillows. Finally I unravelled it - three pillowstightly rolled in a draw sheet! Where were the pillow cases?

Another pre-war facet of the Linen Room was the monthly ward 'Crockery Day'. Once a month, the Linen Room Sister visited every ward, where, laid out for her inspection, was every single item of china, glass or cutlery that was on that ward's official list. Breakages were reported - and when I was training paid for - and Sisters ordered replacements weekly. The crockery day insured that every ward was fully equipped, but it too has long gone. One of my friends, recently a patient in hospital, was offered a boiled egg for breakfast with the information that there were only seven egg cups in the ward!

Clearly, duties in the Linen Room were changing in 1945. My first morning, Sister told me that there was a shortage of laundry workers and that she generally gave the sorters a hand. The wards were still issued with linen bags marked with the name of the ward. Each bag was tipped out onto the floor, the various items, sheets, towels etc. separated and foreign objects removed. Just what nurses in a hurry could send to the laundry was unbelievable - anything from surgical instruments to a bed pan. One of the workers told me she would never be surprised to find a baby!

My second year of training I worked in the Nurses Sick Room. Among the patients was a Senior Private Staff Nurse. I thought she was very old, she was probably 40-45. She was also vain and thought nobody knew that her teeth were false. At night she secreted them under her pillow. There was a lot of fuss one morning, a senior surgeon was coming to see her, I gathered that, incredible as it seemed to me, she had once been his girlfriend. All her bed linen must be changed. Next - the teeth were missing! She insisted I must have gathered them up in the bottom sheet and sent them to the laundry. At this point Sister came on duty, I was soundly rebuked and a message was sent to the Laundry. The sorters were alerted and one of the workers shaking the pillow cases shook out the precious teeth, put not under the pillow, but into the flap turned in at the top where they had stayed when the case was taken off the pillow. That had been twenty years ago, only now did I appreciate the value of the sorter.

A current feature of the Linen Room was the 'Bundles for Britain' sent from America! Practically every afternoon Sister and I would tackle one of the crates awaiting attention. One was entirely full of pillow cases, some new others used, all in good condition. Another was full of men's pyjama jackets - not all the sort to appeal to the British working man, but all suitable bed wear. The funniest was full of corsets! It seems odd, but a lot of thought had gone into them - every shape and size. Tights had not been invented, nor as far as we were concerned, nylons either for that matter. Returning from an air-raid shelter to find one's home vanished, how did one keep one's stockings up? If one had nothing, would one waste one's coupons for suspenders?

I've often wondered if the women of England ever adequately thanked the women of America? Where did they meet, those women - were they similar to our Women's Institutes - and asked each to bring a pillow case to the next meeting? Perhaps they met at somebody's house? That box of corsets should not have come to a hospital, but I could imagine what a boost it must have been to those valiant cockneys always ready for a laugh, who ultimately received it with joy as well as thanks.

Pre-war London Hospital Christmas's were stereotyped. The two senior housemen, one for the east and west wings, were provided with Father Christmas outfits complete with beard. To each were allotted two fairies, preferably rugger players, in complete fairy outfit - and a train of other housemen in assorted fancy dress.

All this was kept in the Linen Room, subsequently collected up by Sister, carefully furbished and put away for the next year.

The Private Staff uniform was also her province. Each Private Staff nurse had two good cloaks, one winter and one summer weight. Rumour had it that fur coats were issued, this before 1914, to nurses going to nurse the Russian Royal family. Private Staff nurses were given a chit to Boyd Cooper's, a West End tailor, for their new cloaks. The old ones were issued to pupil midwives to wear on the district. Finally the machinists let me try to emulate their skills. All ward linen, name of ward and date inscribed in red stitching copperplate - it looks so easy, mine looked like a five year old's first attempt at signing his name.

Up to 1939 all 'The London's' staff accepted that though there were adequate baths, everybody must wash and clean their teeth at the wash-stand, complete with jug, basin, tooth bottle and glass found in every bedroom. By 1945 the wash-stands had gone, but there was nothing in their place. On every floor there had always been Shampoo Rooms with big wash basins, a hollow stopper, about eight inches long and no grid over the hole the water went down. There was a notice on the Shampoo Room doors, 'Not to be used for tooth cleaning!' Where were teeth to be cleaned?

I had been to a theatre, came in at about 11 o'clock in the evening, went to the Shampoo Room to clean my teeth under running water and dropped my two newly acquired false ones - of course they went down the hole! Three years at Merrymeade had taught me a lot. I crawled under the basin and unscrewed the vent. Inserting my finger, it reminded me of midwifery - I found my plate jammed across it - completely immovable.

At breakfast next morning I saw the senior Assistant Matron and told her, most apologetically. Halfway through the morning, I received a message - Matron wanted to see me. I waited about ten minutes and was then told Matron had been unavoidably detained. Would I go to my room and wait until I was sent for. That seemed to me excessive. I was the first to admit I was in the wrong but to be taken off work like that was most unusual - was I to be dismissed?

My dental plate was awaiting me in my room, with an admonishment. The plumber could do no better than I, and had had to saw the pipe through! Finally Matron was ready to see me. When she told me that I was to become one of her Assistants, I said I thought that I was about to be dismissed. The saga of my teeth hadn't even reached her!

CHAPTER SEVEN

MATRON'S OFFICE

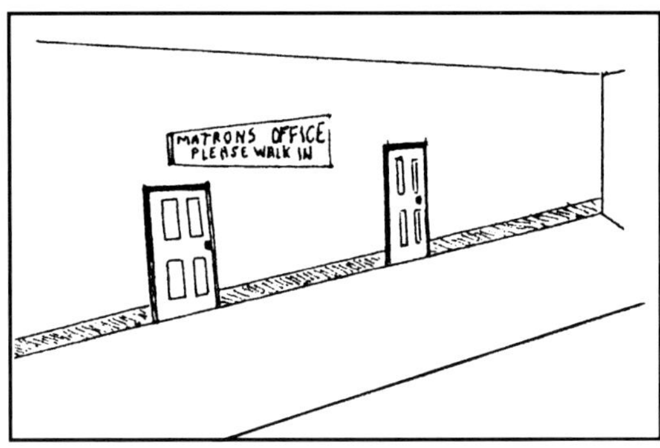

Until the end of the war - 1945 - trained nurses were probably the cheapest, as well as the most efficient, managers available. Specialised training for women was only in its infancy. Consequently, many Sisters held non nursing posts. Six were in charge of the Nurses' Homes and Kitchen. Two ran the Laundry, the junior had a medicine trolley and dosed the workers, a hard working, contented body of men and women, with tonics, cough medicine and the like. Another, called the Housekeeping Sister, was in charge of the Resident Doctors' Hostel and generally mothered the Medical Students. Those doing midwifery, the 'Midder Boys', had a sitting room in which they waited while on call - this was one of her special charges, to be kept supplied with vital stores and dealt with tolerantly after end-of-course parties. She even had to supply tea every day for all the students in the Operating Theatres. Two Night Sisters supervised the army of cleaners, the 'Night Scrubbers' who from 11 o' clock in the evening to 5 o' clock in the morning cleaned departments, offices, corridors and stairs, practically everything but the wards. 'Matron's Office' i.e. Matron and her Assistants were in overall charge.

The era of the trained, other than nurse, professional was just beginning. For many years Private Staff Nurses at The London Hospital had been able to avail themselves of a three month course of massage managed by Sisters. These Massage Nurses commanded a slightly higher fee when they were used to give massage to their private patients. They were also used in the wards as ordered. The London Hospital's Physiotherapy Department went back to before the war and the School of Physiotherapy was well established. Miss Reynolds' vision of the School having at its head a doubly qualified Sister Physiotherapist was never to materialise. The Xray

Department had been run by a Senior Sister, a dragon so fierce that rumour had it that she had been moved to 'Xray' as the only place where she would never come into contact with probationers. Her successor was replaced by a doubly qualified Sister Radiographer and the Radiography School followed. The hospital's Swimming Gala, always held in September, concluded with a fancy dress parade - a skit not a race. In 1948, with the National Health Service three months old, a group of young Sisters came as the 'School for Sisters'. Arrayed in the pleated skirts and blazers of the Physiotherapy and Radiography Schools, their finery was made from old blue uniforms, instead of the physiotherapy and radiography brown or green.

Though her reign had been brief, the first 'Lady Almoner' had been appointed in 1909. Now as 'the Almoner' she reappeared, together with the Dietitian and Occupational Therapist, each with their quota of students. Wardens replaced Home Sisters and Domestic Supervisors took over the supervision previously given by Ward Sisters as well as the general cleaning.

The office itself had been moved. The old one, a spacious suite overlooking the garden at the western end, had housed the two Sisters and secretarial help necessary to run the 200 strong private nursing staff as well as the other administrators. The only external telephone was in a cabinet, similar to a public call box and in one window there was a wash basin where 'Boots', the junior Sister, could refill the ink wells from every desk and wash the slates on which were written the daily staff moves. Matron's Office opening off this was connected with the front desk - Boots - with a horrible internal speaking tube. A further couple of offices lay beyond Matron's and tucked away were two cubicles known at the Green Boxes where the Sisters in charge of allocation worked.

The post war one, the old Samaritan offices, faced the Whitechapel Road at the eastern end. Matron's Office, the inner sanctum, was at one end and the main office at the other, both with doors opening on to the corridor. They were connected by an internal passage off which opened a small office used by the senior Assistant Matron and a secretary's office. There was ample filing space throughout and a plentiful supply of telephones. Outside the main door hung an eye-catching notice **'Matron's Office, please walk in.'** And they did! The volume of traffic in and out of 'the office' was enormous. One welcome casualty of the war was the 'Leave of Absence Book'. Every member of the Nursing Staff had one, there were different coloured bindings for Sisters, Staff Nurses and Probationers. In theory, in it was entered the length of time the owner had spent out of doors every day. In reality, every day - or night - off duty or for trained staff, half day, day or weekend off, had to be entered and the book brought to Matron's Office by the ward or departmental Sister. It was then initialled by Assistant Matron or occasionally Matron herself, and put for its owner to collect, by 10 o'clock at night for day nurses and 1 o'clock in the afternoon if on night duty. Another custom that had been dropped was the 'Dinner List'. Every Ward Sister, as soon as she finished serving her patients dinners had to fill in and sign a form stating that the meal was satisfactory and deliver it to 'the Office'. I once wrote that the meat was tough and inedible. Half an hour later Matron sent for me - it was not for me to pass adverse criticism! The Sister of every ward or department where student nurses (the term 'probationer' was dead) worked still had to report to the Sister in charge of allocation everyday.

When, my newly acquired Blue Belt spanning my waist, I finally reached Matron's office, Miss Alexander, with the able assistance of both Miss Annie Harris, now Principal Tutor, and Miss Ceris Jones, was reorganising nurse training. The Study Day System had just been introduced. This demanded close co-operation between the Sister in charge of allocation and the teaching department. In addition, Ceris was supervising the installation of a more modern method of record keeping - the Kardex system.

Of the other Assistant Matrons Miss Catherine Walker, nearly due to retire, was in charge of the trained staff. Miss Phyllis Stanley, having taken a year's Administrative Course at the Royal College of Nursing, would replace her. Miss Mabel Billington, who had been in charge of The London Hospital unit at Chase Farm throughout the war, looked after the remnant of the Private Nursing Staff and there was a junior Sister. I was to keep an eye on the domestic staff and the laundry.

Another imminent change was the upgrading of senior staff accommodation. The ground floor flat in the Old Home, where Miss Luckes had died, had long been used by the two most senior Assistant Matrons. Now 40 Newark Street, a terraced house with three floors each consisting of a large front and small back room and a basement kitchen had become available. Ceris, Annie Harris and I were each to have a floor. In the course of furnishing we were told we could choose our own sitting room carpet. For some unknown reason we visited the Works Dept singly - there was one nice carpet - and a few others. Ceris was the most senior, I also regarded her as a guest to be treated with courtesy, so I for one did not choose the best. Perhaps nobody did! The Works department staff were as permanent as the nurses - presumably they had their own priorities They had known me for twenty years, Annie for ten, Ceris possibly for two. Whatever - by the time we moved the carpet was firmly in position - on my floor, but nobody minded. The scheme was a great success, with all the advantages of living out added to those of living in.

Before the war, there had been small Annexes at Reigate for both men and women and convalescent homes at Mitcham, Morden and Felixstowe. Now there was the Annexe at Brentwood and another, mainly for orthopaedics, the Zachery Merton Home, at Banstead. Both the Reigate homes, Fairfield and Croft, were functioning and the Herman de Stern Home at Felixstowe had been reopened. The pattern was that on Wednesdays an Assistant Matron visited Banstead and both the Reigate Homes and on Fridays Brentwood. To this were added first The Hora Home at Woodford for elderly and long-term convalescents and ultimately Hayes Grove, a home for elderly sick nurses. Though our visits there were sporadic we also had an interest in Queen Mary's Maternity Hospital at Hampstead, which became part of 'The London's' School of Midwifery in 1945. One or another of the Assistant Matrons visited the wards of The London Hospital daily.

My first summer 'in blue' I had worked briefly in 'the Office'. It must have been at the height of the holiday season; one of my friends was 'Boots', I was even more lowly! Since then the atmosphere had changed. Miss Ford, in charge of the Private Staff had ruled with an iron hand, but there was a self-indulgent streak in that generation. I can remember stray cups of tea being brought in by a nurse from the Receiving Room (Casualty). Miss Alexander was just the reverse and expected her own standard from her staff. Not so much as a tumbler existed anywhere and if even a glass of water became vital it had to be borrowed from the nearest ward. An air of professionalism prevailed which was certainly conducive to work.

I did not find being a 'new girl' easy. I was aware that I was not the colleague Miss Walker would have chosen and 'Please walk in' was a challenge! The Assistant Matrons gathered in Miss Walker's office at 2 o' clock every afternoon for briefing. One day in my first week, 'Boots' was off duty, I was left to mind the Outer office. The door opened and a senior porter ushered in an undistinguished looking woman. He evidently saw my look of surprise and announced, 'Mrs Roosevelt' - it was the First Lady of the United States - the President's wife! Nobody had thought fit to warn me that she was expected. I was left with the impression that I should have handed her over to Miss Walker to escort to Matron!

As a junior Night Sister, it had been my privilege to underline in red ink the headings of the senior Night Sisters report! I now found that these, after Night Sister had reported to Matron, were left in 'the Office'. When for the first time since my arrival we entered a new month, Miss Walker gave me the month's bundle and a ball of string and instructed me to bore holes in them and finally tie them up! Just as in 1938 I had felt there must be something better to do after fifteen years nursing than clean instruments, I was sure twenty years experience could be put to better use than boring holes in foolscap. In due course I gave them to the most junior of the secretaries, who dealt with my correspondence, and left her happily stringing the reports together. Unfortunately, Miss Walker found her so occupied. 'Did I not realise that the secretaries were PAID and could not be given such work'. I ventured to suggest that a typist was probably paid less than either she or I. I was never again given the night reports to deal with, but many years later was staggered when Dame Phyllis Friend told me that she had been given them to do when first she came to Matron's Office. I wonder - who did them in the years between?

One of the nicer of my daily visits was to the Laundry. It was no longer run by Sisters - Carrie was in charge. Carrie was a comfortable, middle-aged woman, who had come to work in the Laundry when she left school at thirteen. One of her early jobs had been to iron Miss Lückes' handkerchiefs - she must have been a treasure even then. She had the whole place running like clockwork. When she retired some years later she was replaced by her daughter - Young Carrie.

One day Carrie sent for me - she never came to 'the Office'. She suspected one of the porters of stealing - by methods I hate to contemplate she had found that before going home at night he was in the habit of rolling sheets round his middle under his clothes. This was quite soon after the war, before theft became prevalent or the unions dominant. This information was relayed to the House Governor, and while the man was met outside the laundry door by police, his home was searched. With everything rationed the temptation must have been great. At about the same time a representative from the local cleaners and dyers brought a cotton suit to Matron's Office. Before being dyed it was a plain white coat and skirt - with the dye the 'London Hospital property' woven into the material - it had been a sheet - was clearly apparent. That was another thief caught. The next was not. After visiting time one Sunday afternoon a Ward Sister came to report that the lavatory seat in one of the patients' lavatories had gone. A carefully premeditated theft.

V.J. Night (Victory in Japan), August 14th 1945, again took me to the gates of Buckingham Palace. Several of my friends, including Dame Phyllis Friend, tell me that they too were among the thousands there. This time I went with a couple of friends, but when the Royals had waved for the last time, the balcony lights had been switched off, the doors clanged shut and the crowd surged homewards, I found myself inexorably propelled in one direction - my companions were borne away in another.

As the Temple Underground Station came into sight I thought that was where I would get a train, but when I saw the queue and remembered how drunk some of my homeward companions of V.E. night had been, I decided I would walk. Along the Embankment, through the City, Aldgate, no longer filled with haycarts, and back to 'The London'. The war was over - we were safe - we were free. It was a wonderful feeling.

In the 20's the wonder of Christmas in hospital had held me spellbound. I recalled the transformation of the wards on Christmas Eve, the candlelit procession singing carols at 4 o'clock in the morning, Father Christmas distributing gifts to the patients, their Christmas dinners, and finally, 'the shows' travelling from ward to ward.

In the 30's as a Ward Sister it became more of an endurance test. Decorations, stockings to be filled as well as gifts for Father Christmas to distribute, and above all catering for patients and an unknown number of visitors. It was customary for Consultants to visit their wards, sometimes bringing their children. Above all, no members of the nursing staff were off duty over Christmas. The patients' care was not in doubt, but to ensure the necessary atmosphere for really ill people and to keep too many nurses happy needed constant juggling. For me the best moment of Christmas was on Boxing Day when, the festivities safely over and the decorations put away ready for next time, I turned the key in the lock of the Christmas cupboard.

By Christmas 1945 the war was behind us. It was a period of austerity - everything that could be was rationed, even electricity was in short supply to be used sparingly, but the bombing was over, the blackout gone and people were being released from the forces. It was my first Christmas in administration and I realised that if Ward Sisters worked hard, so did Matron's Office'. Carols had been brought forward from 4 o'clock in the morning to late evening. Miss Billington, was the conductor. It was customary for two senior Sisters, of whom from then on I was one, to lead the procession - the ability to sing was immaterial, it needed people who could be trusted to set the pace and head in the right direction.

Toys were not rationed, just in short supply and difficult to get hold of. In the course of the year a small hoard had been built up, sufficient to provide for the sick children spending Christmas in hospital. When in the course of Christmas Eve the cupboard was unlocked, it was bare. The entire stock had been stolen. How that piece of information became news was a mystery, but on the six o'clock radio news it was announced, just a bare statement 'The toys to be given to the sick children spending Christmas in The London Hospital had been stolen'. In Matron's Office we did not even know of it. The first response was about an hour later. A man carrying a box, holding a small boy by the hand walked into Matron's Office. He handed the box to the child who gave it to me - "For a sick child " -, the train set he was to have been given the next morning. I could have wept. Next came two teenagers, they had come by bus bringing their model yacht, a treasured possession. By the time I had got back from Carols the trickle had become an avalanche. The pile had been moved from Matron's Office to the Board Room.

A late arrival was the Matron of a Children's Home bearing, I felt, the best of the things destined for her own brood. She was obviously relieved when I explained we had already received more than enough and needed little persuasion to re-pack her basket.

Well after midnight I answered the telephone - the duty officer from a Midlands Police Station - "What should be done with a parcel left with him?" A clockwork duck had taken his eye, I suggested that perhaps if he put it on the doorstep facing South it would lead a procession to us! After that I for one did just briefly get to bed. My last contact was at the Front Entrance as I came on duty next morning, the owner of a small toy factory, he had driven out there and brought to us his remaining stock.

By this time the press had picked up the story and the finale was on Boxing Day when a press photographer arrived, I spent best part of the morning in the Board Room with two or three convalescent children and a couple of student nurses surrounded by toys. By the end of that incident I really did understand the truth of '...it is more Blessed to give than to receive'.

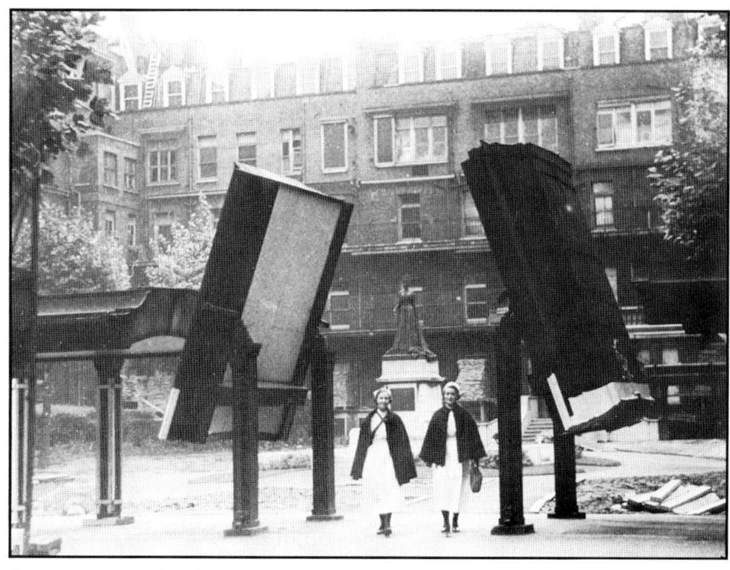

Covered way, centre portion tilted open during wartime, London Hospital quadrangle, October 1939

CHAPTER EIGHT

STAFFING V TRAINING

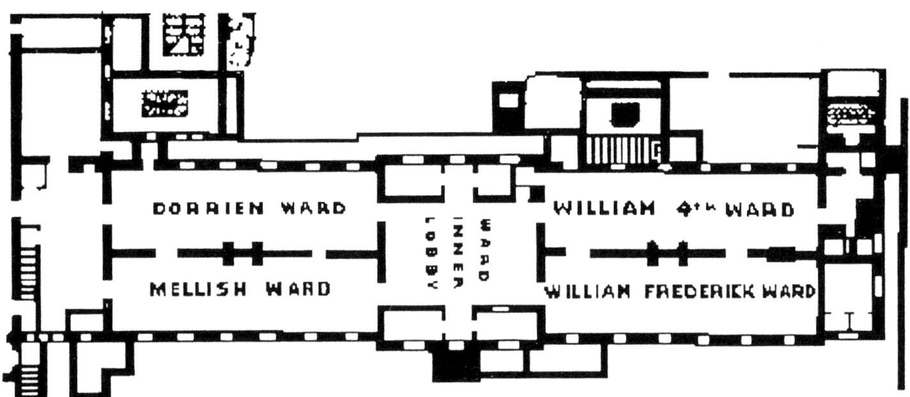

When 'The London' was built, nursing as a profession was not even a dream. The pattern of staffing would have evolved from the structure of the wards. Each ward unit was built round a central lobby. Two double wards, each sub-divided, contained, by the 20th Century, 56 beds in four sub-wards each containing 14.

Originally, one Sister was in charge of the whole unit and there she lived. As a newly appointed Ward Sister I found, in one of my desk drawers, an inventory of ward furniture. It included:-

Sister's Sitting Room
1 writing table
1 occasional table
1 armchair
1 upright chair

Sister's Bedroom
1 bedstead
1 wardrobe
1 dressing chest
1 wash stand

I have been told that the first duty of a night probationer of that era was to clean the patients' bath in readiness for Sister's use and erect a corridor of screens across the lobby so no patient could catch a glimpse of her in her dressing gown.

In the second half of the nineteenth century a Sister was appointed to each ward. 'Sister's bedroom' became the sitting room for the additional Sister and both slept in the Nurses' Home. The off duty time of the two alternated so that by day the unit was never left without a Sister.

By the twenties, the four year period of training was well established, three years as a probationer and the fourth, compulsory, as a staff nurse, either in hospital or on the 'Private Staff'. Every ward had two staff nurses who throughout their year alternated twelve week periods of day and night duty.

Nurse training, as it developed, was of the apprentice type, with the bulk of the teaching in the Ward Sister's hands. In Miss Lückes' lectures she stressed the importance of what she described as 'intelligent obedience', but throughout her training the probationer was learning to accept increasing responsibility. It was probably the sub-division ward pattern that had led to the 'pro-staff' system.

The 'pro-staff', (probationer staff nurse) marked by a shining S pinned on her apron, was a third year probationer who for six months, three on day and three on night duty, was junior staff nurse in a sub-ward.
A staff nurse worked in the other sub-ward and only when the Sister was off-duty did she assume command. From the responsibility angle it was a perfect system, on completion of her six month pro staff period, the third year nurse was well prepared for the responsibilities of her fourth year, but by 1945 the training angle was gaining in importance. Six months, a sixth of the whole training, was deemed too long to spend in just one type of experience. Miss Alexander reduced it to three, with the further three elsewhere. It was a more important shift in the balance of training than was readily apparent. For the first time academic knowledge had taken precedence over practical experience - the acquisition of managerial skills was diminished.

The opening of the link block wards in 1962 altered the ward bed pattern. The sub-wards no longer existed, the pro staff, and the 'S' itself became a thing of the past.

Not only must every ward be adequately staffed, with first, second and third year student nurses to meet the requirements of its patients, but every student nurse must have a well-balanced training. This was the problem with which Ceris was juggling, the eternal battle of staffing v training. Pre-war training had run on stereotyped lines. Every probationer started in a general medical or surgical ward. It was unusual to remain in any ward longer than four to six weeks. Three months of each year was spent on night duty, the first one beginning at three to five months. Three months in 'Out Patients' usually followed. There was practically no full-time theatre experience, but as the gynaecological, ophthalmic, and septic surgery wards all had their own theatres and tonsils were removed in Aural Out Patients, most nurses gleaned some knowledge of the theatre. With four children's wards, eighty cots, every nurse had good paediatric experience, but most missed out on one of the specialities such as ophthalmic or ear, nose and throat.

Now the emphasis was on following the requirements of the General Nursing Council. In addition, a new system of record keeping was being introduced. 'The London's' method was probably unique. On entry every trainee was issued with a stiff backed, black notebook, the 'Black Book'. In this every day of the next three years had to be accounted for, but the owner must not write in it - this was done by the ward or departmental Sister.

On the last day of the month the book had to be put open on Sister's desk together with a slip of paper, its corners neatly cut off, e.g.

Sophia Day Probationer
September 19th - 30th
Please Sister.

Sister duly entered and initialled the entry and the books were posted in Matron's Office letterbox. They were returned to the Dining Room next day. Duplication or omission of any date was marked in red ink, evidence of the owner's carelessness. What no probationer, or student nurse according to her date of training, ever knew, was that the 'Black Book' was handed in, not to be checked, but for its contents to be copied into the appropriate register. In other words, the 'Black Book', compiled by its owner, WAS the record. Both register and 'Black Book' were now in the process of replacement by a single card to be kept up to date by an additional secretary.

The Private Staff Nurses, in the wards between cases, had always been available for emergency help either in a ward crisis, or general shortage, such as a flu epidemic. Normally, they, like the Sisters, came on duty at 8.30 after 8 o'clock breakfast. When being used as 'pairs of hands' they, like the staff nurses, were deployed on 'seven o'clock duties' following a 6.30 breakfast. With the running down of the Private Staff this was no longer possible and was another factor to be taken into account when staffing was planned. Allocation must have been easier when the whole hospital was under one roof. Now both Brentwood and Banstead had to be staffed and the experience gained there included in the whole.

A small room across the corridor from 'the Office' had been allotted to 'the Kardex' and there, on a trolley beside the secretary's desk, stood the cabinet housing the whole. For every student nurse one card, so filed that it could be studied, or written upon, without removal. The card was headed with the full name, age, education and any previous experience of its owner. The middle section summarised the information the Black book had contained - details of experience gained - day duty - night duty - holidays and sick leave, accounting for every day of the training. The bottom gave experience in weeks so that one could see at a glance what had been done and was yet to do. A photograph of the student was attached.

A new secretary had been appointed solely for the Kardex. Miss Flora Abraham, like Matron's Secretary, was resident, living in the Nurses' Home and having her meals with the Sisters. This meant that she could, when necessary, have the afternoon off and spend the evening working with the Sister in charge of allocation. Evenings were the only part of the day relatively free from interruptions. The Kardex was Miss Abraham's pride and joy. She rarely actually saw any student nurse and she certainly never set foot in a ward, but she seemed to have the record of every one of them in her mind's eye!

The Weekly Study Day System had been introduced in August 1945. The 9 o'clock in the morning lectures that I had accursed so whilst in the Private Wards were a thing of the past. The new system gave all students sixteen days each year, spaced at weekly intervals, in the Class Room. Each course was held twice a year. The study days began at 9 o'clock in the morning, ended at 4.30 in the a fternoon and were followed by the student's weekly day off duty. First year classes were on Mondays, with Tuesdays a day off. Second year classes were on Fridays with a day off on Saturday. The third year nurses, who were valuable in the wards at weekends when trained staff were off duty, attended Wednesday classes and were off on Thursdays. From the allocation angle this meant that for thirty-two weeks of the year half of the student staff was attending classes for one day of each week. During their Class Days, student nurses could not be put on Night Duty neither was it feasible for them to be working in Out Patients or the Theatres, experience in which was now compulsory. It was a good system with many advantages, but meant that allocation was a challenge and like a jigsaw puzzle that one never quite completed.

Until the war the probationer was given a full calendar month's holiday on completion of training, before returning for the compulsory year as a staff nurse. This was now optional. 'The Month', as it was known, remained for those returning to the staff.

In the early days of nurse training The London Hospital certificate was the owners only proof of training. Miss Luckes seems sometimes to have added a note on its reverse side so that it served as a testimonial. In the twenties the hospital certificate was complicated. It covered the nurse's practical work and her 'conduct'. There is reason to suppose that 'excellent' was only written against 'conduct' if that nurse had never once in her whole training been late for 6.30 o'clock breakfast!

The certificate also covered the theoretical side and was signed by Medical and Surgical staff concerned. The hospital final examination was marked and prizes were awarded to those obtaining the highest marks, 'prize probationers'. Nothing had ever been made of having gained one's certificate, but at the turn of the century the 'prize pros', with their parents, were invited to the Medical College Prize Giving, held in the College Library, where their prizes were awarded in the same way as those of the medical students. When Sir Frederick Treves presented the prizes he added a gift of his own, to the year's winner.

Now, the hospital certificate was awarded only to State Registered Nurses. The certificate itself was a smaller, simpler document and every nurse was also given a hospital badge, which previously had to be bought. The badge had been introduced in the thirties by Miss Monk, every one was inscribed and it is recorded that one of the earliest recipients was Queen Mary, President of The London Hospital.

Miss Alexander had instituted not a prize giving, but an annual presentation of certificates and badges, held in the Medical College Library. In March 1946 Queen Mary herself presented the certificates and badges to nurses who had completed their training in 1945 and also to Physiotherapy and Radiography students who had qualified during the year. It was a splendid occasion, Her Majesty spoke to each nurse individually. The Laundry had excelled itself, Nurses wore their uniform with pride and the medical staff in their academic robes added colour to the platform.

Miss Alexander had made great efforts to improve living conditions in the Nurses' Homes. What had been the Nurses' Sick Room, by the back gate, became the Nurses' Dining Room. Strangely, after various vicissitudes, by the 90's it is again being put to that use.

Like everybody else, Ceris and I had found the Nurses' Home extremely cold that winter but electric fires were being installed. Also every bedroom in the Nurses' Home was being supplied with a bedside light. Twenty years earlier we had discovered that with a piece of flex and some string one could utilise the centre light, so that one could read in bed, but it was a nuisance to dismantle it before going on duty!

I watched the Kardex system being implemented with great interest. Ceris and I had become firm friends as well as colleagues since my return to 'The London'. It was obvious that she would not remain as an Assistant Matron for long. In May 1947 she left to take up an appointment as Matron of Westminster Hospital. I was very sorry to see her go, but delighted to think that I was to be in charge of allocation.

CHAPTER NINE

PROFESSIONAL LIFE

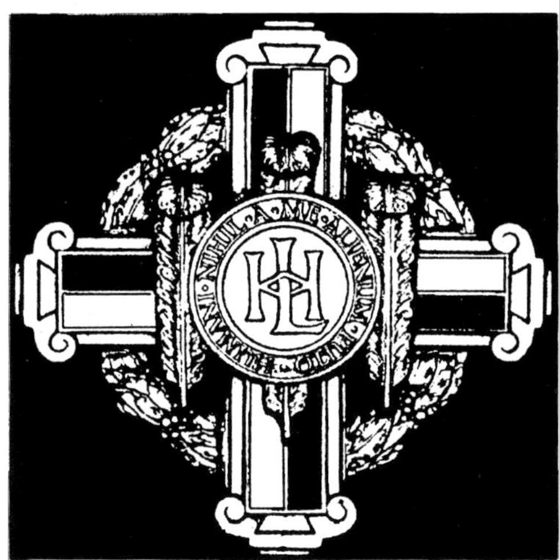

Work 'in the Office' fell into a regular pattern. Against the daily 'staffing v training' background were a number of annual events, moving from one to the next, the years slipped by with incredible speed.

My professional awareness dated back to my days as a holiday Sister, when a meeting of the Association of Hospital Matrons was held at 'The London'. Two other holiday Sisters and I were detailed to assist generally. It was evidently beyond the scope of the Catering Department, so we spent the morning preparing tea, among other things there were 200 bridge rolls to fill! We directed the guests to the Medical College Library on arrival and afterwards marshalled them to the Dining Room for tea. I remarked to a somewhat forbidding looking female that we were passing the statue of Queen Alexandra, 'the only one in the country'. She enquired 'was I sure' - it transpired that her previous guide had told her it was Queen Victoria! In case help was needed we were to attend the meeting. We climbed to the balcony at the back of the Library and amused ourselves counting the numbers brave enough to wear hats of neither black nor navy blue - hatlessness of course was unthinkable. It was the first time I had ever thought of nursing beyond 'The London'.

Miss Monk, then Matron, founded The London's own professional organisation, 'The London Hospital League of Nurses' in 1931. A professional organisation meant nothing to me, I regarded 'the League' as an activity only for those who had left. Early 'League Days' culminated with a Dinner in the Medical College Library. As a Ward Sister, leaning over Harrison balcony, I watched the League members, they must have brought a change of clothes with them, streaming out of the Old Home and realised I was missing something.

By the end of the war we were more aware of professional organisations, there were the College of Nursing, the National and International Councils of Nurses.

League meetings featured largely on our year's programme. Whether it was one's Saturday on or off duty was immaterial, League Day was a long, heavy day. No matter what time the meeting officially began, erstwhile Senior Sisters, sure of a suitable welcome, would be looking in on 'the Office' on arrival well before it started.

The war curtailed the activities of the Professional Organisations. One of my Sister Tutor Course friends had been to an International Congress of Nurses in Paris just before. The first post war one was in the United States. Miss Clare Alexander and Miss Phyllis Stanley were among those who attended. Miss Mabel Billington and I went to the next one - in Sweden. A number of overseas delegates came on afterwards to visit London before returning home. Two of them, whose hospitality both Clare and Phyllis had enjoyed, stayed at 'The London' and a special post Congress Dinner at 'The London' itself was arranged. It was to be a splendid occasion - a small commemorative gift, a vase of authentic pottery suitably filled, marking the place of each female guest. Not all the guests invited had responded to the invitation and it had been assumed that silence meant refusal. Dinner was about to be announced when we realised that there was one extra guest! Like most people from large families, I had been brought up on the F.H.B (Family Hold Back) principle, but Mr Bowler, the Catering Officer, wouldn't hear of removing my place name and managed to juggle in an extra place. The only comment made was by the nicest of the Americans who remarked loudly, "You've got no flowers". She was to reply to the Chairman's speech of welcome - she had discussed if beforehand with me, so sitting back complacently I was shattered by her opening, "Sir Mann!" English is a foreign language even to Americans!

'Billie's' and my excursion to Sweden had a bad beginning. We had booked accommodation in a hotel within walking distance of the Conference Centre. It was evident from our reception that something was wrong - how much so was revealed by degrees. The agent was not there and our bookings did not exist. Our hosts were deeply concerned and an hour later Billie and I were offered hospitality by the Matron of a large mental hospital twelve miles away - not what we had planned. Used as we were to the restrictions of a Nurses Home, the inaccessibility of a Mental Hospital, locked as securely as any prison, was new to us. Our resourceful hostess had the answer - she gave each of us a master key which would open every door in the hospital. The first time we returned at midnight Matron herself was with us and showed us her own unconventional method of gaining entry, even so, a twelve mile bus journey whenever we sallied forth was somewhat daunting.

Professionally I remember only a session on training within industry, referred to as T.W.I. - of universal interest regarding the ever increasing numbers of extraneous people involved in hospital.

In the course of the week I met a charming Swedish Nurse who told me she was hoping to come to London the following year. Thinking of devoting a half day or so to showing her the sights I said let me know. A year later I had a letter from her, giving the date of her arrival and saying she could stay for a month! Clare laughed when I showed her the letter and said that would teach me to be more careful in speaking to foreigners. Billie had friends in Yorkshire, a retired Londoner was running a guest house in Devonshire, between us we arranged a good programme. Severely rationed as we were we were touched at the gift she had brought us - a whole ham! Asked if there was anything she particularly wished to see she completely floored us - a visit to a London Pub! Not only had neither my friends nor I ever set foot in one, we were not sure what constituted one nor which of our men friends, conversant with their local, would be good guides. There was no question of unescorted women going to a pub.

In addition to professional matters Clare tried to widen the horizons of her staff in other directions. She arranged for Constance Spry to come and speak on 'Flower Arranging'. Before the war, the junior Night Sister was responsible for keeping fresh flowers on the war memorial in the Front Hall. The Assistant Matrons dealt with the flowers in the Hospital Chapel, open always and used on Sundays, which amounted to 'doing the Chapel Flowers' as one of the regular chores for one's Saturday on duty - no imagination required.

There was also an attempt to create interests for the ever increasing numbers of Lay Staff. With that in view the first Security Officer organised a Flower Show. Clare said that each of her assistants was to submit an entry. Our only source of flowers was Covent Garden entailing an early morning visit to the market. I, however, had recently became non-resident and there was a copper beech tree in the garden - I had already experimented with beech leaves and hydrangeas and on my last visit to Brentwood had noticed a magnificent display round the hospital entrance. Rather than toil to Covent Garden I rang my friend, Hillman, now the Head Porter at Brentwood, and asked if half a dozen or so hydrangea blooms would be missed - he promised to put them on the van. Complete with beech leaves, I left home half an hour early the next morning, found my bucketful of hydrangeas and selected a vase from the Chapel store! I then went off on the Banstead round to be greeted on my return by my colleagues who said it was grossly unfair - not only had my entry gained the first prize but an extra one for originality, and it hadn't cost me anything!

Presentation of Certificates Day was another of the big occasions. Selection of the date and speaker were not my province - at our level, checking the names and dates of every nurse was the first step. Phyllis Stanley and I did this jointly - as full name and dates of training appeared on every certificate and badge, it had to be done well ahead - a time consuming exercise.

There are said to be three steps up any professional ladder - first one's shoes are cleaned, next one's letters are written and lastly one's speeches composed. One year the certificates were to be presented by a high ranking army officer. A nice young man, whose level was presumably comparable to my own, was his speech writer. Together we produced a lovely speech - all the details accurate, everything apposite included. All other details covered, I took my place on the platform confident that nothing - this time - could go wrong. The speaker stood up - I was all attention, but within a couple of minutes Dr Harry May, the Dean of the Medical College, sitting beside me murmured, 'He's muffing his lines'. Who could have anticipated that he would have come without his spectacles! What a lot of effort wasted, but as he shook hands with each entrant he gave the impression that this was the most exciting thing that had ever happened to him. The nurses were unanimous - he was wonderful. They would probably not have remembered the speech anyway.

Spectacles featured in another incident a year or two later. There was a brief period, I don't know how it was discovered, when Ceris could see better through my spectacles than her own. I was having a serious discussion with the father of a student nurse when the newest office recruit came bounding out of Ceris's office tweaked the specs off my nose with, "Matron must have your glasses", and tore them off. The man I was talking to was fairly stunned and finally came out with, "This is a hell of an office". How I agreed.

Christmas, with all that it entailed, loomed largely over a relatively long period. One year Miss Alexander decreed that every patient should have two visitors to tea on Christmas Day. When I said something about this to one ward Sister she said, "Washing up for ninety at tea time may be your idea of a Happy Christmas, but it isn't mine!" She was surprised to see me on Christmas afternoon, but I was whisking off my sleeves - I had gone to wash up.

State examinations were another recurring event, though as the number of Tutors increased our involvement with the examination itself lessened. The day the results came out was another story. As a member of the General Nursing Council, Miss Alexander came back from a meeting bearing the results the night before the candidates were notified so we were at least primed.

Those of us who were General Nursing Council examiners were allowed time away once a year - it seemed to work out at one time in the London Area, next further afield. When first I became an Examiner, for the Preliminary Examination, the candidates had vivas as well as a practical part. On one occasion during the war one of the Medical Examiners was in naval uniform, young to be examining. One of the others said that surely in war conditions everybody should pass. The naval one was adamant that nobody had told him to lower the standard. Having risen from a 'Preliminary' to a 'Final' examiner, I was once greeted by a candidate - did I remember examining her for 'her Prelim'!

We were singularly fortunate in our relations with the lay staff. The porters in particular were all friends. The daughter of friends of mine was a physiotherapy student. Her father visited her when she was warded with some minor ailment and arrived at the front door just as Miss Alexander returned from a session at the General Nursing Council. He told me afterwards - she had handed her coat and brief case to the nearest porter who was as gratified as if she had been royalty. I tried to explain to him that Matron was probably rated slightly higher than even the Queen.

I was once taking two of my young nephews out. My sister was to put them on to a Green Line bus which stopped at 'The London', where I would retrieve them. The coach stopped and an indignant passenger who had seen the boys handed over to the conductor informed me that they'd been put off at Mile End. Before embarking on a search I alerted the Front Hall porters. The Head one, complete with gold braid, did not hesitate - he would join in the search and actually it was he, clutching one of the boys firmly in each hand, who delivered them to 'the Office' before I'd wended my way back from Mile End! It was typical.

Year by year the numbers of additional 'professionals', employed to relieve the Nursing Staff of non-nursing duties increased. One of them was a head Domestic Supervisor; responsible for all non nursing staff previously under Matron's jurisdiction, she came under the aegis of the House Governor. The first one, a very superior personage, was to be attached to Matron's Office for a week or two while she found her feet. It was a period of mutual enlightenment! Forty years ago a hospital was not the employment centre it is today and it attracted employees who liked people. The four Assistant Matrons between them represented fifty to sixty years of 'London Hospital' experience and there were not many of the lay staff that one or another of us did not know.

The newcomer had obviously never before come into contact with trained nurses. It took her a few days to accept that we really did know most of the people coming in and out of 'the Office'. Her voiced surprise at our unfailing politeness left us speechless!

The Social Secretary was another innovation. Until Miss Reynolds became Matron, such recreational activities as there were for the Nursing Staff had in been in the hands of one of the Assistant Matrons. When I became a Tutor in 1938 Miss Reynolds forced me to become secretary of the newly formed Sports Club. This lapsed during the war and, much to my joy, was restarted with a Social Secretary, based in the Luckes Home, responsible not only for tennis and swimming but for all recreational activities. Miss Stone was an established figure for many years and as counsellor and friend was invaluable to each succeeding intake of student nurses.

There had always been a Nurses Library. One wonders by what twist of fate it had become the province of two senior Out Patient Department Sisters! Two evenings a week, the two Sisters from the Light Department opened the Library, it had professional books as well as a fictional section, in the Luckes Sitting Room. The library was now moved to the main building with a part-time librarian in charge. A rota of volunteers took trolleys of books to the wards for the patients' benefit. Mrs Hargreaves was another of our good friends, she always saw that we, in 'the Office', had any book we particularly wanted!

The hospital hairdresser had been functioning at the Annexe at Brentwood during the latter part of the war. She, too, was established in the Luckes Home. She, again, was wonderful. There was always time for Matron and her Assistants to be 'swept-up' at a moment's notice when the occasion demanded!

CHAPTER TEN

THE APPOINTED DAY

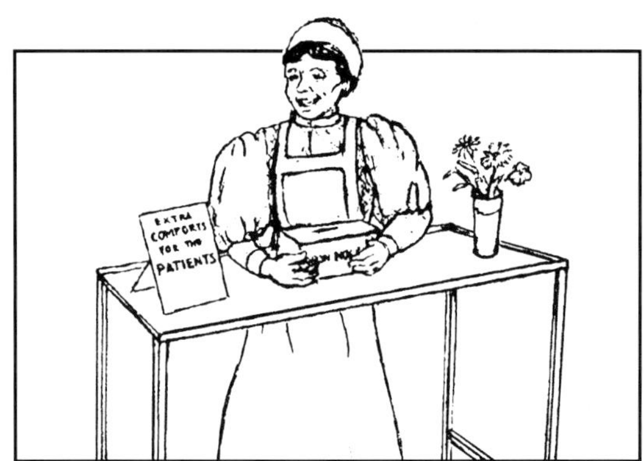

Except that no longer would a nurse with a collecting box stand at the ward door as visitors left, July 5th 1948 was just like any other day. For two hundred years 'The London' had lurched from one financial crisis to the next. Now the voluntary system was replaced by the National Health Service. The guiding principles of John Harrison, the founder, in 1740 had been:-

1. The charity was free to the sick poor.
2. It was entirely dependent on voluntary contributions.
3. Doctors gave their services.

When Sydney Holland, later Lord Knutsford, the 'Prince of Beggars', first came to 'The London' in 1895 it was at a very low ebb. By the turn of the century, thanks to him, 'rebuilding' of the hospital was in full swing.

By the twenties finance was again a problem. The hospital was still free to the sick poor, but only just. Patients provided their own butter, tea and sugar, no small item for the really poor. At the end of each visiting time a nurse stood at the ward door with a collecting box, 'Extra Comforts for the Patients', even those two or three pennies must have been an effort for some. As probationers we wondered what were extra comforts. As Sisters we found out. It comprised such essentials as dressing gowns and pyjamas, neither of which was included in the ward inventory. They were more necessary then than now as relatively few patients had either. I once enquired of the wife of a newly admitted patient if she would be bringing his pyjamas and was told, " 'E just slips in", as indeed did many others.

In the thirties a Pay Office was opened and Pay Office Clerks visited the wards to assess what small contribution a patient could make towards his upkeep. As a Ward Sister I used to waylay them. They always agreed when I suggested that no contribution could be expected from, for example, a man who had a wife and two small children and who would never work again.

From the time we entered hospital economy had been instilled into us. 'Poor people have denied themselves to help the hospital and you are throwing it away', we would be told if we had left a tap dripping or an unnecessary light on. I once suggested to a student nurse who had left an electric fire on overnight that it was her father's tax that she was wasting. She replied happily, "I don't think he'd mind." Nursing staff salaries were paid quarterly and every quarter Lord Knutsford wrote a letter to 'The Times' - "The London Hospital had no money to pay its nurses", contributions poured in.

Throughout the war some state support had become essential - the voluntary system was doomed. In 1942 the Beveridge report on Social Insurance Allied Services was published. Beveridge considered that 'for every citizen there is available whatever medical treatment he requires, in whatever form he requires it..........................." There was to be a complete comprehensive medical service free to the patient.

There was no place for private nurses in the National Health Service. The London Hospital Private Nursing Staff had been steadily running down ever since the war ended. They were a great loss, particularly in the midwifery field. Generations of mothers had benefited from 'monthly nurses'. The last remaining ones were much in demand. I once took a telephone call from a would-be patient. "If", she enquired, "we had a baby in ten months time, could nurse so-and-so come? Can I book her tentatively now?"

Only State Registered Nurses must now be employed - the hard core of Sisters who had never bothered to register could do so - or leave. The last two Sisters of my generation who wanted to stay on, delayed registration as long as possible. It seemed expedient that they should not take the examination with 'The London's' current entry. Attired in white overalls, they presented themselves at another Centre for their ordeal, only to be confronted by Miss Ceris Jones, who by some curious coincidence had been allocated to examine there. I never heard the views of the victims, Ceris did not enjoy the experience! Both did pass. One of my set never did become State Registered. There was plenty of work available, but as she found to her cost, the nurse companions of elderly ladies have no pension rights.

I had been fifteen when the first war ended. The generation of spinsters resulting from the deaths of a million young men was roughly ten years older. For thirty years they had carried nursing - and teaching - and provided the stability from which my generation had gained so much. Now the voluntary system they had served so well was over. They, themselves, were approaching retirement. They had worked in nursing and non-nursing posts throughout the country. At The London Hospital they had formed the backbone of that unique institution, the Private Nursing Staff. In her wisdom Miss Lückes had early instituted a pension scheme for nurses. At a minimum age of forty-one and after twenty years service the nurse was to be entitled to a Pension of £60 a year. Ours was one of the last sets to be included in that scheme. As we had 'signed-on', we were given our choice, join the Superannuation Scheme, or remain in the hospital's own. At the age of twenty, twenty years is a long time. Few of us looked that far ahead, most had remained in the old scheme. Until the outbreak of the second war all 'The London's' trained staff had led well ordered, comfortable lives. They had known nothing other than the petty restrictions in force and, on the other hand, the standard of service provided for them was unbelievably high.

That between-war generation have my utmost sympathy. Cheated by war of normal fulfilment, that of wife and mother, they had worked extremely hard for relatively low salaries. Taken for granted all their working lives they retired unsung to genteel poverty, if not absolute penury. Up to about ten years ago people would say to me, 'but you must know of a retired nurse who would be glad of a comfortable home in exchange for just keeping an eye on - ?'

She or he would probably have demanded full nursing care, not to mention housework and cooking.

That September the Assistant Matrons themselves participated in the Fancy Dress Parade at the Swimming Gala. Matron's Office never closed and it was well known that Miss Alexander allowed neither eating nor drinking in the office. If a glass of water was essential it was borrowed from the nearest ward. Heavily made up, bejewelled and unsuitably shod, they carried placards:-

Civil Servants
Office Hours 10am - 4:30pm

Closed for Lunch
12 - 2pm

Closed on Saturdays,
Sundays, Bank Holidays
and Saints Days

The last one carried a fully equipped tea tray, but all this was fantasy - not fact.

Happily engrossed in allocation, the appointed day made no immediate impact on me, though the nursing staff in the wards were delighted to abandon the visiting time collections.

The arrangement had always been that requests for emergency repairs outside normal office hours went to Matron's Office. It was about 9 o'clock one night when the man in charge of the boiler house telephoned - could an electrician come and change the light bulb in the boiler house. Like the nursing staff, the maintenance staff was an established force, we had all known one another for many years, so I said, "Come off it Bill, where is the bulb in your pocket?" His reply was, "But Sister you don't understand, I am not allowed to touch anything electrical." So an electrician had to be brought from his home to change one single electric light bulb. That was the first time I realised that we were no longer part of a voluntary hospital.

Miss Mary White, who had come into the office when Ceris left, now visited the Laundry. A Union representative asked if he could talk to the Laundry workers. He did so and they were quite happy to join a Union and pay their weekly dues. Six or eight weeks later one of the workers asked Mary White, "When is the outing?" She went on to explain she had paid every week. To their way of thinking you only ever paid in if you were subsequently to draw out. So, by degrees, we did come to realise that things had changed.

I was sad to learn that Ellen had died - returning from a visit to her sister she had collapsed in the lane leading to Merrymeade where a passer-by found her body. At Miss Alexander's suggestion I went in uniform to her funeral. This was from her sister's house and the coffin was screwed down after the funeral party assembled. I was acutely conscious that it was not what the Ellen of whom we had been so fond would have wanted for me. As a mark of respect I was invited to lead the company in prayer. In the dark watches of the night one's inadequacies rise up to confront one - that is one of my rccurring ones. It was a foggy afternoon. As the small funeral party, Ellen's family, Winnie the cook and I trailed through a vast impersonal cemetery I was filled with regrets - why had I never told her how much we appreciated her - one of the war's many unsung heroines.

CHAPTER ELEVEN

A CHANGE OF MATRON

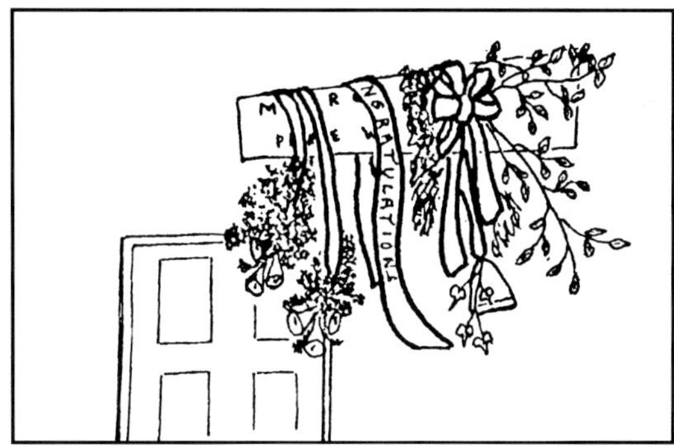

The announcement of the engagement of Sir John Mann, Chairman, and Miss Clare Alexander, Matron, took The London Hospital by surprise. The next morning coming on duty, I found Night Sister, at the top of a pair of steps removing from the 'Matron's Office Please Walk In' sign the decorations draped over it by the 'on-call' Medical Students.

The Assistant Matrons should not have been surprised. About two years previously the Luckes Home Sitting Room had been the scene of an innovative party. When 'Auntie B' had returned from Warley, the magic touch had no longer been enough for the Sister of a Children's Ward - she must be a Registered Sick Children's Nurse - so Auntie B became a Home Sister in the Lückes Home. She gave those post-war student nurses the same love that she had lavished on a generation of East End babies, and they gave her a leaving party. Not only had there never before been a leaving party for any Sister, but this was the first time any man had penetrated to the Lückes Home Sitting Room.

The organisers were Kira Claringbold (Holt) and Unity Urquhart (Kingsmill) whose parents in the States had sent a wonderful food parcel, hence the name, 'The American At Home'. Amongst others they had invited Sir John Mann as Chairman, Captain Brierley, House Governor, Dr Clark-Kennedy, Dean of the Medical College and Miss Alexander and senior nursing staff. Miss Alexander presented the tea service which was their farewell gift. For me, there was, however just one salient point to the party - in the course of it, how I do not know, I realised that Sir John's interest in Clare was not purely professional. When the opportunity presented itself I suggested, had she ever thought of marrying the Chairman. Two years later when she told me she was leaving to be married, she added 'You can't say you were surprised, it was your idea'.

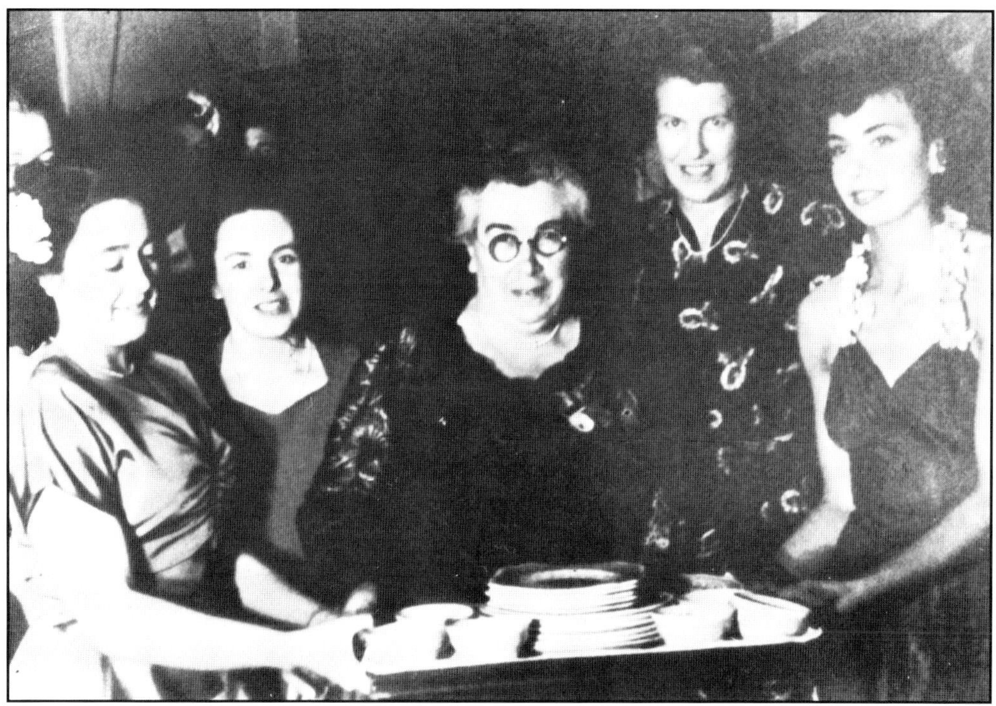

The American at Home, presentation to Miss Leslie. Centre Miss Leslie, Miss Alexanrder on her left.

In her time as Matron, Clare had carried 'The London' through the war and into the National Health Service. She had revolutionised 'The London's' nurse training after its long period of virtual stagnation. She was an active member of the General Nursing Council - with an ever increasing work load she had never spared herself. It was a state that could not have been maintained, but all of her assistants were devastated to think of 'The London' without her. I once overheard two nurses discussing her as Matron, one of them said, 'I could die for her'. I could appreciate that sentiment, she had been a joy to work for.

When Phyllis Friend (Dame Phyllis Friend) joined the Matron's Office team Clare told me, 'Miss Friend will go far, you are to teach her everything you know'.

Miss Alexander's leaving was characteristic. Until mid morning she had been in her office as usual - we simply failed to realise that she had gone - for ever. Sir John had invited the whole of Matron's Office Staff to a party at the Savoy that evening - there he announced that he and Clare had been married that afternoon. Clare told me that she was surprised that I had not worked out the plan of events!

The appointment of a new Matron took time and the successful candidate would have to give due notice to her current employer. There would be a gap of several months. As holiday Sisters we had learnt that every well run job goes on its own momentum for at least as long as it takes to pick up the threads. To some extent the same applied but we were 'ships officers' without a captain! Naturally we took a keen interest in Clare's successor. Ceris, as Matron of 'Westminster' was the obvious person but happily settled there would she want it? I was moved to say to the House Governor of one applicant that I knew that I could not work for her, so should be leaving if she were appointed, to which he replied that he would come with me!. Miss Reynolds had been appointed just before I had returned as a Tutor in 1938. Junior as my role was, I had seen enough then to realise how essential the loyalty of her staff was to any newcomer and I was determined that whoever she was, Clare's successor should not suffer in that way - as it was we all welcomed Ceris wholeheartedly. Miss Gweneth Ceris Jones was uniquely qualified, trained at St Thomas's, Assistant Matron at 'The London' and Matron of ' Westminster'.

When it came to her first ward round as Matron Ceris was smitten with nerves - so I went with her to Croft, literally on the doorstep of Matron's Office. Croft was quiet apart from patients, not a sign of life anywhere. The student nurse behind the curtains around one bed had evidently heard the door open - a face peered out, registered abject horror and withdrew. Talking to the nearest patient, Ceris and I waited. The student nurse, a junior one, collected herself - came up to us - and curtsied! It dawned on me that just as I had been, the girl must have been at a convent school. The curtsy could even have been a nervous reaction, but Ceris was shattered. It would have taken very little to reduce us to helpless giggles. As it was, when we were safely outside again Ceris enquired, surely you don't teach them to curtsy?

All royal occasions were suitably marked, Coronation Day June 2nd 1953 was no exception. Ceris, as Matron of The London Hospital, had a seat in Westminster Abbey - this necessitated an early start. When, in a lovely golden coloured dress, with matching handbag for the prescribed sandwiches, she reached the Front Hall, she was greeted by a guard of honour. With a true sense of occasion, Night Sister had amassed every available night nurse to speed their Matron on her way.

Every member of the hospital staff had an extra day off. Those able to have the actual day largely set off early to get a place on the route of the procession. The whole world saw the Queen of Tonga braving the rain in an open carriage. The London Hospital nurses came back cold, wet and bedraggled, full of their adventures, to be revived by hot soup specially laid on by the Catering Department.

Television was still in its infancy - but a set had been hired for every ward so that all patients well enough to do so could share this momentous event.

There must have been many like myself who had not seen television before.

Ceris was also to have attended the funeral of Queen Mary, but the previous day she was unexpectedly summoned home owing to her mother's serious illness. I was deputed to ring up Marlborough House to give her apologies. Whoever answered the telephone said would I go in her place! As Assistant Matrons we had our own code of honour - everything else being even we drew lots for any unexpected bonus - but was this one? It was reluctantly decided that I had just been lucky. This was mid morning the day before the funeral and a black outfit was essential!

My brother lived in Hove. I knew his wife had a black coat, but this was a lot to ask. However Lucy rose to the occasion - she packed up her coat, took it to Brighton Station and put it into the hands of the guard on the 1 o'clock London train. I was waiting on the platform when the train drew up at Victoria, and complete with coat crossed the road to Gorringes where I bought a black hat and a jumper! With a little help from my colleagues my black outfit was impeccable next morning when I made the fourth of 'The London's' contingent, Sir John and Lady Mann, Captain Brierley and me - we went in a hired car to St George's Chapel at Windsor. Afterwards we saw all the Royal Family even the Duke of Windsor. Finally Sir John took us to lunch at the Savoy. When we reached the entrance to the Dining Room, Sir John requested a table for four, the head waiter replied, 'Yes My Lord' That really did make my day.

Queen Mary had been a regular visitor and we knew her well. Her progress round a ward bore some relation to any administrators round. She was capable of asking what do you keep in that cupboard? She loved babies and the maternity wards were always included in her itinerary - on one occasion she remarked, 'If the wall of the ward balcony were to be white washed the ward would look much lighter.' The day before her Majesty's next visit Miss Elizabeth Major, the Superintendent Midwife, came to the Office - the wall had not yet been whitewashed! The Works Dept tackled it immediately and as the Queen stepped into the ward the next day she commented on the improvement.

The Queen's first visit replacing Queen Mary as Patron was eagerly anticipated. Sir John Mann was a wonderful host and talked gently throughout. Her Majesty seemed to enjoy the tour. One of the regular guests at Royal visits was Lady Hudson, previously Viscountess Northcliffe, after whom Mary Northciffe ward had been named in 1920 - on this occasion I escorted her to the Boardroom where tea was to be served and told her she was to sit next to the Queen. She would have made no comment had it been Queen Mary, but the Queen was evidently different, 'not the little Queen'.

Lady Hudson was obviously as able a conversationalist as Sir John, I heard her opening remark as to the health of the children.

Between five and seven o' clock on Friday evenings an element of peace descended on 'the Office'. There had always been a slackening of pressure over weekends - no chief's rounds, no theatre lists, even medical students disappeared. Traditionally, before the war, Ward Sisters were off duty from 1 o' clock on alternate Saturdays. As every bed curtain in the hospital was changed once a month, Sister's departure was the signal to change the curtains, previously folded, on one side of the ward but even so, the tension lessened.

With the enormous increase of auxiliary staff this was even more noticeable. The keys of a number of departments were kept in Matron's office and one after another would be handed in - the department closed until Monday. The Physiotherapists and Radiographers, like the Nursing staff, were vital. We had become accustomed to extra qualifications, it had even extended to nursing staff e.g. the Sisters in the Children's Wards were R.S.C.Ns and Sisters coming into Administration had taken a year's course at the R.C.N. Now we had to learn to work with Almoners. The Samaritan Society, founded by Sir William Blizard in 1791, its motto 'Take care of him', had always dealt with that aspect of the work. The link between that department and the Nursing staff had been two Sisters and transfers to Annexes and Convalescent Homes ran seemingly like clockwork. Private Staff Nurses, in between cases, were available for use as escorts as required. Convalescence was now the province of the Almoners Department and there was no longer a private nursing staff. Nurses in training never had been used as pairs of hands, but bearing in mind the requirements of the G.N.C. every student's experience was carefully monitored. Special Ambulance nurses therefore became a necessity - there were to be three of them. My first foray into the art of interviewing involved one of them. I chose what I considered to be the best of the applicants, only after she had started work did the Cashier's Office point out that she was over seventy! I had not asked her age.

Before the war most of our patients were local. As a Ward Sister, I can remember the admission on a Sunday afternoon of a small boy whose parents had brought him from the Midlands on a 'cheap day excursion' - in due course he was collected in a similar way. Ambulance journeys then were almost entirely to and from 'The London's' Annexes and Convalescent Homes. Now there seemed to be patients requiring transport over long distances. The Almoners had developed a cumbersome 'ambulance - train - ambulance' journey. The patient - and escort - were taken to a main line station - travelled by train and were met and taken either home or to another destination. A crowded train must have been an ordeal for any patient ill enough to need an escort and no fun for the escort either. It was an unpopular chore! One Friday morning a young almoner presented me with an itinerary she had booked - to Wales - for Sunday! I pointed out that the Ambulance nurses did not work at weekends and that there was nobody else - she simply could not grasp that nurse escorts were not inanimate objects, waiting for use. Having declared the journey could not be cancelled, she finally, at Matron's suggestion, escorted the patient herself. There was never another Sunday journey!

The rule was that all letters coming to Matron's Office were answered the day they were received, but there was always paper work on which to catch up over the weekends. A brief history had to be written on every student nurse whether she completed her training or not, it was there for reference purposes. Until the introduction of the Kardex System, these had to be laboriously copied into the appropriate 'Volume' - now safely deposited in the Archives. We had a dictaphone but weekends were subject to endless interruption.

One Sunday afternoon the door opened and a man ushered in two small children. The rule 'no visiting by children under twelve' was still in force. 'They won't let me take them in to see my wife, I can't leave them outside - you can have them' and he was gone! I was alone, but mercifully neither of the children seemed perturbed. Father came back at the end of Visiting Time to find them, shored up by Registers, sitting at desks, paper caps on their heads! With paper, pencils and a telephone apiece we were playing - not 'Doctors and Nurses', but 'Sisters'. It had fairly wrecked my afternoon! Another time a woman came in, edged close to me and said, 'I'll be safe with you'. It wasn't my afternoon that was wrecked that time. Borrowing a nurse from the nearest ward and assuring her that by saying, 'Hold the line' or 'Take a seat' she could cope with both telephone calls and enquiries, I took my visitor to the 'Receiving Room' (Casualty). Hours later a harassed Receiving Room Officer came to tell me that he had managed to resolve the situation. He was too polite to tell me what he really thought.

The funniest intrusion of all my years was on a weekday evening. We were heavily engaged in some imminent social occasion. Matron's Secretary was also in the Outer Office so it was to her that the old man made his request - had we accommodation for relatives of dangerously ill patients? This was not a Matron's Office responsibility - one of us would have queried it, but Miss Clarke took it at its face value and within a few minutes she very cleverly obtained the required address. Thanking her and clutching his scrap of paper, as he edged out of the door he came out with, 'I knew you'd be able to tell me where I could get a bed the night before the Cup Final!'

Another of our weekend problems was the Private Wards. Their bed occupancy was in the charge of a Secretary, dragon enough to have been mistaken for a pre-war Sister. She was responsible only to the House Governor, provision of the Nursing Staff was all we did, but Miss Butler went home on Friday evening and reappeared on Monday morning. I was waylaid by Colonel Cahusac, the Deputy House Governor, one Monday morning with, 'This is where we disappear into the sunset'. He and I, in charge over the weekend had, at the urgent request of a Consultant, admitted an emergency into a bed booked for Monday morning! Rare as it was, the reverse could happen. A woman carrying a suitcase walked in about 4 o' clock one Sunday. Her admission had been planned in readiness for surgery on the Monday - and there was no bed! That really was difficult.

Night Sister, left with the information that a patient with a wholly unpronounceable name was expected, was confronted in the middle of the night by a family, man, woman and child, without a word of English between them. She put the woman into the bed, got a cot sent up for the child and tucked the man up on a settee in the waiting room. Morning - and an interpreter - revealed that he was the patient!

Matron was away and the House Governor on duty the Sunday that Night Sister reported that there had been a flood in the maternity wards - they had let the steriliser boil over. The Board Room directly underneath had only just been redecorated - Yes - it had seeped through. I went to look, 'seeped through' was an understatement! I left a message with the front hall porters, would they let me know as soon as the House Governor crossed the garden from his flat. I was back forty years - remembering that to be shown, rather than to discover, damage goes a long way towards to lessening its impact. What could be said?

In no circumstances did we talk to the press. Only when no member of the House Governor's staff was available were such calls put through to Matron's Office - and even then they must be parried. A very persistent reporter and I had had a long discussion on a Sunday afternoon - finally he had enquired, 'who is - at this moment - in charge of the hospital'? I had to admit that probably I was and got the reply, 'you can't be as stupid as you sound'!

CHAPTER TWELVE

WHERE DID WE GO WRONG?

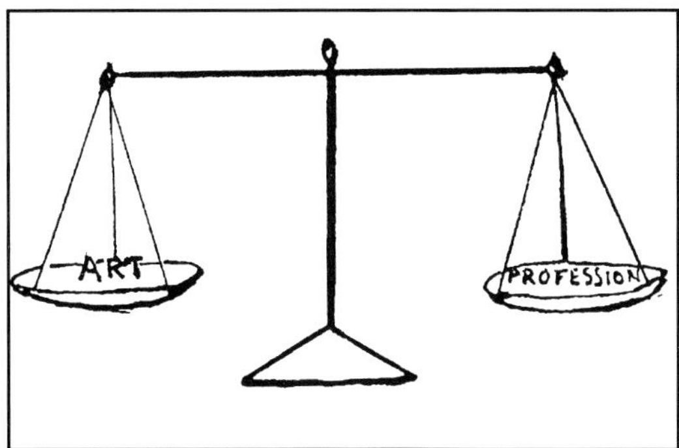

"I shall hold you personally responsible if ....' Irate consultants were one of the occupational hazards in Matron's Office, but this was different. The senior neurosurgeon was threatening, 'provide a special - or else'. We were just embarking on a 'pre-intensive care' period that would culminate with the opening of an Intensive Care Unit.

Surgery was moving on and demanded a new level of highly skilled nursing care. It was a challenge that could and would be met but this was 7 o'clock in the evening. The surgeon was threatening dire consequences unless the patient on whom he had just finished operating was provided with a 'night special' - a nurse entirely to himself. Strange as it may seem, at that hour it was impossible to increase even by one the number of night nurses about to come on duty.

Every weekend the Ward Sisters drafted the off-duty time of their nursing staff for the coming week. Every morning they provided a list of their staff for that particular day and between 9 and 10 o'clock, the Sister in charge of allocation compared the two - linked with the night staff worked out a month ahead. At that time, in emergency, a day nurse could be asked to be on night duty that night. Free from 1 o'clock, it was reasonable - but not 7 in the evening. When planning allocation the aim was to provide one or two extra nurses every night, these could be used as required. The Private staff, always a final fallback in emergency, had ceased to exist in 1948 and the 'bank nurse' had not yet come into being, there was no redress.

The change in post-operative care was noted, both day and night Sisters included pending operations in their daily reports and we in allocation were on the look out for them. As a longer term measure, a system of 'internal night duty', whereby the 'Special' as opposed to 'General' wards arranged that the last few days of every student's experience was spent on night duty in that same ward was introduced. There were several advantages, for the patient, there was continuity of care. He already knew his nurses. For the student, each one had experience covering the whole 24 hours. It had always seemed unfair that some had experience of a particular speciality, e.g. gynaecology, on night duty only - indirectly the system shortened the usual twelve week period of night duty.

But what of that particular night? One of my colleagues in charge of allocation at another hospital solved the problem by becoming the special herself, much to the consternation of the consultant who visited the patient concerned at about 10 o'clock that night!

I once had a difficult interview with the Mother of a child in one of the Children's Wards. She was complaining bitterly about the number of nurses involved in Tommy's care. It was useless to go into the number of hours in a week divided by the hours of a nurse's working week or to explain that even nurses must have meal breaks, she was not interested in the mechanics. She felt it would be better if Tommy had two nurses covering the twenty-four hours! She would have approved of the Private Staff regime. Another nurse and I once spent six weeks nursing - in a hotel - a child with scarlet fever. We worked a twelve hour shift, 1 o'clock to 1 o'clock. That way each had about half of the child's sleeping and waking hours. The Mother looked in occasionally and the General Practitioner at intervals - apart from that neither the child nor the nurses saw anybody else at all!

We were facing a familiar problem - was nursing an Art or a Profession? Miss Lückes, founder of the London Hospital Nurse Training School, was in no doubt. In the Preface to the 2nd edition of her book, 'General nursing', in 1898, she writes:

"There is a real danger in the present day that the fact that nursing is an ART may be lost sight of; and work which affords scope for the exercise of some of the most beautiful qualities of which human nature is capable may thus be degraded into a mere profession."

In the first chapter she reiterates:

"People too frequently forget that nursing is an Art. This fact must be remembered and nursing must not be regarded merely as a profession".

Way back in the twenties when all nursing staff were single and resident, we worked a 65 hour week. The only ancillary staff was one wardmaid. The nurse in training therefore had much more time in which to practice the Art and there was no indefinite line of demarkation as to who did what. Hours of duty ran with split second precision, nursing care was equally meticulous. To quote Miss Lückes again:-

"People learning to play the piano do not enjoy practising scales and five finger exercises but they know that the object they have in view is well worth the trouble".

Turnover of patients then was much slower. 'A hernia' remained in bed for three weeks, even a clean appendix ten days. Although there were seriously ill patients in every ward, we were in effect largely nursing well people in bed. Many patients were transferred to Annexes before they were up - to all intents and purposes all our patients were bed-ridden and every single one received attention to pressure areas. The night nurses were responsible for the morning washings and though many patients would have washed themselves their backs would have been 'done' - and any other pressure areas if necessary. The buttocks were rubbed with a soapy hand - rinsed, dried and powdered or rubbed with spirit. Every bed had a draw sheet, which was pulled through leaving an absolutely crease free surface below the patient. Ill patients would have had attention to pressure areas during the morning, for the rest there was a quick round immediately after dinner - the back was rubbed, the draw sheet drawn through again and, as a frill, the 'red', the blanket covering the foot of the bed, given a quick flick with a clothes brush before the patient was left for an after dinner nap. Beds were made again between 5:00 and 6:30 after the evening washings. I remember the day in 1927 or 28 when the second wardmaid was introduced into the ward team! From then the two ward-maids would take-over sweeping and washing-up of breakfast which had always been the nurses first task. This change in no way affected nursing care.

I have vivid memories of the first surgical dressing I watched. I had been trusted to prepare the trolley - Sister was to change the dressing. First the patient was prepared - the bedrest was let down and the patient comfortably settled - the bed clothes were turned down - minimum exposure was essential. 'Binders' were used for all abdominal wounds - the era of sticky tape was yet to come - so the binder was unpinned and finally Sister went to scrub-up - the preparation itself was an Art and afterwards the patient's back was done and draw sheet pulled through as the clean binder was put on. The whole procedure was only a few minutes - the Art of nursing at its best.

The war had brought endless changes, new drugs, new methods of treatment requiring new skills. The nurse of the fifties required new technical knowledge, but the basic art remained. Early ambulation revolutionised the time spent in bed, though it had to be remembered that the patient who sat up in a chair was not necessarily well, he did still need attention. The time patients spent in hospital was reduced - the pressure on the nursing staff increased. By the fifties the old fragmented care was changing to a more individual approach, one nurse responsible for the whole toilet, this in its turn has given way to the 'named nurse' largely extolled in the popular press today.

In my Final State Practical Examination, in the late twenties, the Examiner demanded, 'Tell me about bedsores'. I started to say I had never seen one - thought that reflected lack of experience and substituted, 'In my hospital we don't have bed sores'. Whatever the examiner thought, it was true. Yet today they are so prevalent that the Minister of Health speaks openly of the need to take action for their prevention. How did my generation come so unwittingly to lay the foundation for this situation? Where did we go wrong?

Bedsteads have changed, so have mattresses. The 24" water pillow placed under the buttocks and so beloved by the patients has become obsolete. Possibly the old red mackintosh sheets were kinder than today's plastics? Assuredly the soft cotton draw sheet was better than today's and the laundry probably used a less fierce form of washing powder. All these can however only be minor factors - meticulous attention to pressure areas was the keynote.

Nurse training was changing - more time was spent in the Classroom, apart from which the hours spent in the Wards were reduced. Bringing the day nurses on duty at 7:30 instead of 7 in the morning was probably the most drastic change of all. Early ambulation added to the confusion. Before the war, the morning routine finished, Sister came on duty at 8:30 to a scene of complete order; I once heard it described as 'every patient's nose in a line with the centre crease of the top sheet'. 'Up patients' could hardly be chased into bed for Sister's benefit, so added to the new disorder, but no ancillary help could replace that lost third of the 7 - 8:30 period.. As Assistant matrons, visiting the wards daily, we were aware of the changes - flowers, taken from the wards overnight were, first, still in the lobby mid morning - and finally not taken out at all. Similarly, Prayers, the landmark marking Sister's arrival, lapsed.

I drew up the time tables for the first ward orderlies. Their duties excluded all nursing procedures, they were, for example, to make empty, but not occupied, beds. Why did we not tackle the problem more positively? Patients fell roughly into three categories; those who required no physical care - by degrees a day room where they could watch television and have their meals ensured that they were not confined to a chair beside their beds. My irate neuro-surgeon would have expected his 'special' to be familiar with highly specialised techniques, the basic needs of the helpless patient remained unchanged - the 'special' would have combined the two. In time this section was dealt with in the Intensive Care Unit, the patient possibly returning to his ward via a high dependency unit. That left those, formerly practically the whole, who required full nursing care, none of it technical - the helpless patients.

I recently asked a Londoner trained in the 60's, could she say, as I had, that she had never seen a bedsore? The few she had encountered marked the trend - why had we not seen it coming?

I was a General Nursing Council Examiner and was examining State Finalists in Practical Nursing elswhere when I received an urgent message that my Mother was dangerously ill. I reached home latish in the evening, Mother was deeply unconscious and had been for some time. Our General Practitioner, a forthright woman with plenty of common sense, blew in after her evening surgery. She was quite definite - there was nothing to be done, she would come again the next day if necessary. All my Ward Sister's instincts were to embark on the routine care of an unconscious patient - my sister seemed appalled - the doctor had been quite definite, so we settled for a night long vigil. By the early hours there was no change, I persuaded my sister to go home and get a little sleep. Surveying the situation I decided to cut off the night-dress Mother was wearing rather than try to get it off. I had the scissors in one hand and a fold of nightie in the other when a voice from the bed said, "Margaret, what do you think you are doing?" When the doctor visited next morning Mother, at her own insistence, was sitting up in an armchair. She made an uninterrupted recovery and lived several years, but the bedsore due to that overnight inaction on my part took a month to heal. The care I should have given to anybody else would have prevented it. That episode is one reason why I am convinced that most bedsores should never occur.

How did my generation fail to notice that basic nursing care was being overlooked?

My sixties trainee assured me that in the Class Room great stress had been laid on 'meticulous nursing care'. The time spent in the Class Room increased, but the Art of Nursing can be acquired only at the bedside - in participation. It is learnt neither in the Class Room nor by observation.

My personal experience of the Art came just before the end of my training, when I had diphtheria, necessitating ten weeks lying flat in bed. Blindfold, I could tell the good from the indifferent, I KNOW that nursing is an Art; it is not just manual dexterity but an intangible something that makes nursing worthwhile.

It must have been easy for the undemanding passive patient to be overlooked amid so much activity, but we were responsible for both patient and student. We should have realised that the experience available to the student was changing. The basic nursing care, previously listed in ward reports as, 'two hourly by day, four hourly by night', was becoming a rarity. The new student, just as she was shown new developments, should have been given every opportunity to participate in it. It is the keystone on which nursing is based and to reach perfection must be done over and over again.

Miss Lückes likened the student nurse to a musician; striving for perfection both need an instrument on which to practice - would one deprive a musician of his piano?

CHAPTER THIRTEEN

THROUGH THE FIFTIES

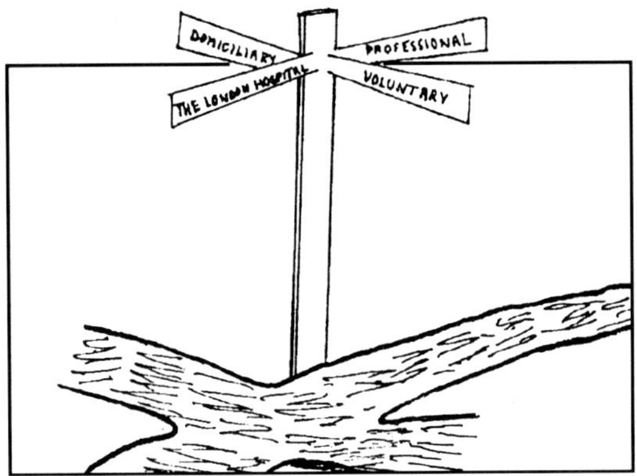

The post war period of innovation was followed by the consolidation of the 50's. Where Miss Alexander had planned Miss Ceris Jones brought to maturity. Nurse training was on a sound basis, good examination results were the norm but change was continuous. We had laughed at the earliest effects of nationalisation e.g. the woman brought to Out Patients by ambulance who told the driver, "We've finished our shopping, now you can take us home" - but the change had already begun. The patient's treatment was his right. Hospital property was no longer sacred. Every member of the staff, whatever his capacity, was affected.

Exclusively involved as I was with the training of the student nurse and ward staffing, it was the change in those young people that struck me most forcibly. My generation had just accepted whatever happened to us, but it was more than twenty years since my training. In the Methodist Church, on the first Sunday of every year, what is known as a 'Covenant Service', a renewal of vows, is held. The opening of the final prayer might well have been the rule of life for The London Hospital probationer signing her agreement, 'I am no longer my own but yours - put me to what you will -'

In the 20's the probationer was marked into breakfast at 6:30 and on duty at 7:00 in the morning, finishing at 9:20 at night. She was told by her Ward Sister, who came on duty at 8:30 at what time she was to have her daily free time, usually 9 - 12 noon or 2 - 5 in the afternoon. There was normally 48 hours notice given concerning the fortnightly day off duty, which began at 7:20 the preceding evening - one's only opportunity to arrange an evening out as a late pass on a day off was regarded as a great privilege. Arrangements for holidays too were hit-and-miss - 15 days for each 6 months worked, but notification of dates given at less than 2 weeks ahead.

Mrs Claire Daunton, when she was 'The London's' Archivist, once asked me what did we do with our evenings. She could hardly believe that one came off duty at 9:20, was marked into supper at 9:30, had to be in one's room by 10:00 and the Homes were patrolled to enforce lights out at 10:30. All too soon it would be 5:45 and the rising bell would ring. Despite all this my generation were courted, loved as much and probably married more than those in the 50's. They had one advantage - during those inter-war years 'The London' had no female medical students to compete for husbands!

The girl of the 50's demanded - rightly - a life of her own. Non-residence for student staff had not yet begun, but residence was more relaxed. One of Miss Alexander's early reforms was the introduction of holiday request slips. I can remember my horror, one January, at finding practically the whole of the summer's second year class was demanding the same fortnight's holiday in August giving as reason 'to attend the Edinburgh Festival'. Fifty - sixty fifteen day holidays could much more easily be staggered over 4 - 5 weeks than a mass exodus.

On one occasion a student nurse returned from her holiday and immediately put in another request for an early date. When asked, she told me, "I've just been away with Daddy and his new wife, and there'll be terrible trouble if I can't do the same for Mummy and her husband." That was my first introduction into the broken home problem - it hadn't happened before the war. Holidays were approximately six months apart, preferably one in winter and one in summer. To have one holiday in early March and the next late September, when overseas travel was still rare, was hardly fair. Clare Alexander and I pondered on the hapless product of the broken home - she said that if I arranged it I would have to cope with the ensuing list of similar requests! Fortunately there were none.

Days off duty also presented problems. 'Weekends' i.e. Saturday off for this week and Sunday for next were much in demand, but the wards had to be adequately covered at weekends. Special occasions such as 21st birthdays we always met but I did resent being regarded as a fool. When one girl put in a request for a weekend for her brother's 21st I remembered having only just arranged one for her own - a date I could check on her Kardex card. I asked her, had she step - or half-brothers - had her mother had one of those rare births of twins born at different dates? My heart warmed to another third year student, a regular request maker, in a real crisis due to sickness I asked would she do one night's night duty in the ward where she was working. Her reply was "You've always given me what I've asked for, I don't see how I could refuse".

Equally, my generation never queried their experience - the post war generation had no hesitation in doing so. Fortunately the Kardex cards provided an accurate record. Some complained of a particular type of work. I sympathised with those who hated the theatres, and was tempted to say, 'Matron did too", rather than point out that it was a General Nursing Council requirement. Occasionally it was the Children's wards that they did not like - one girl told me she did not know what to say to children. Having had a mother that people in child trouble were apt to turn to - in the 1919 'flu epidemic' we had a motherless toddler whose parents we scarcely knew until such time as his father could make arrangements for him - I was slow to realise that an only - or youngest - child might well have never encountered anyone under five years old.

More often it was third year nurses, afraid they were going to miss out on a particular type of work in which they were interested who came to see me, for example, "I've not yet done any Chest Surgery". They were always reassured to find exactly what they had had so clearly recorded - and sometimes see my pencilled entry on their next move.

Not all change was for the better. The use of first names crept upon us - insidious, inexorable. I rang up a ward asking for a message to be given to a Student Nurse Blank. The junior student nurse answering did not hesitate, there was nobody in the ward by that name. I queried, 'Miss Penelope Blank'? Light dawned, 'You mean Penny'?

I was not alone in fighting that one. If Matron was not available, consultants coming to see her usually saw the Assistant Matron they knew best. I had been at Warley with the Alan Perrys, who had become my personal friends, so it was to me that Mr Perry complained of the free use of first names in the Theatres. 'They all call one another by their Christian names'. He enlarged on this theme, 'You know, Margaret, its not right'. I agreed - and avoided saying, 'no Alan it is not!'

Nursing was rightly ceasing to demand the whole time devotion that it had always exacted. Non residence for student staff had not yet become an option, but life in the Nurses' Homes was becoming more independent. Some members of the trained staff had husbands and a mortgage, though not yet a baby, like other people.

Reports were a recurring problem. In theory it was so simple. The Ward or Departmental Sister was given the form with the name and relevant dates filled in, she wrote a few lines, the nurse then signed the statement that she had read the report and the form was returned to 'the Office'. Matron saw all reports and at stated intervals throughout their training saw all student nurses. She was available at any time to any nurse wishing to see her and a bad report generally meant that Matron would like to see the nurse concerned. On one point, however, Matron was adamant. She would not see unsigned reports or their owners. I often thought how much easier the old verbal 'Sister to Sister' hit and miss method must have been! Sisters were busy and difficult reports, in particular, tended to be left. The nurse completed her experience, had gone on holiday or on night duty or Sister would bring the unsigned report to me, saying Nurse So-and So will not sign this. All students finally accepted that nobody was asking them to agree with the sentiments expressed, merely that they had read them. Ceris, as Matron, had an excellent relationship with the student nurses. She had a warm outgoing personality and they appreciated her concern. They knew she would understand their problems - provided the report was signed.

Transferring the students to Brentwood and Banstead made allocation more difficult. Student nurses, particularly in their first year, were happy provided they were not separated from their friends.

I once visited a Pharmaceutical firm and watched the girls working on a conveyer belt: **A** held the bottle for the tablets to drop into, **B** added the wisp of cotton wool, **C** screwed the stopper on and so on. The man in charge assured me that provided they were in the same place, with the same friends on either side, they were perfectly happy. Much the same principle worked with transfers to the Annexes. I always got from each set a list of who was friendly with whom and moved them more or less together. An irate father once rang up and said his daughter was miserable - I had sent her to Brentwood parted from all her friends, she was so lonely and unhappy she would probably leave. I got out my list and pointed out that his daughter had been transferred with nurses X, Y and Z, said to be her friends. He said they were not her friends - I next sent for the set leader. With considerable embarrassment she admitted that they had decided amongst themselves that we should probably separate them and had produced what they thought a successful false list. The father did have the grace to apologise! I always had a degree of sympathy for student nurses going through a sticky patch. I had only once in my training encountered a bully. When, on my 'day off', I told my father that I was not going back to hospital, he pointed out that they had never wanted me to start and of course I could come home, but it was two years of my life wasted and what did I intend to do. Confronted by an angry third year student nurse who had stormed into 'the Office' saying she was not going back to such and such department again I put to her my father's question, 'What will you do tomorrow' - and it worked.

Social life too moved on. The pre-war 'Sunday School treat' sort of Christmas dinner on Boxing Day, the sole pre-war nurses festivity, was replaced by a Nurses Dance. One Christmas, Matron thought this would be easier to control if every nurse came to the office to collect her tickets on which was to be written the name of her partner. Three friends came in together - their partners were Messrs 'Smith, Brown and Jones'. I said they couldn't possibly leave out Mr Robinson, hadn't they a friend who could bring him. At least we all understood one another.

The House Governor, Captain Brierley, and his staff always supported nursing occasions, educational and social. He always expected us to be able to put a name to every nurse, no matter how glamorous the transformation from uniform. At one dance he asked me the name of a young woman that I had definitely never seen before! We nearly had a Matron's Office meeting on the dance floor - finally the House Governor tackled her partner - a medical student - he had crashed in with an outside girlfriend for a dare!

The major social events were not easy. The wards had to be covered as usual by adequate staff but nobody should be disappointed. For us they entailed a degree of actual preparation too - our attendance was obligatory. On the night of one Nurses Dance we had finished decorating the hall - the swimming bath floored in - in readiness and were just saying that we, ourselves, would have time to change in comfort when Matron's buzzer rang. Being at that moment nearest to it I answered. Captain Brierley was with Ceris - it was the Christmas after the Queen's first visit. "Had anybody written up that visit?" It transpired that he wanted an account of it. That was no problem until I enquired "When - " and he said, 'by nine o'clock tomorrow morning'. One of the aphorisms of our day was that 'The London expected the impossible and got it'. I had just two further queries - how many words - and would his secretary type it. As I closed the door I heard his comment "She didn't bat an eyelid". That was something someone somewhere had forgotten or overlooked - I never knew. Captain Brierley however always gave credit where credit was due, it was late, very late, by the time I reached the dance, but as I arrived he came to meet me with, "You've earned a drink!"

It was in the 50's that the surplus woman disappeared for ever creating an entirely new problem. She had long carried teaching, nursing and the care of the young; in various guises from companion or lady-help to maids of all descriptions she had supported the old. My great-grandmother celebrated her 100th birthday in 1912. Lovingly cared for by two daughters, one single the other widowed, she died a year later in her own bed. Whenever my grandmother took me to visit her I was given tea in the basement kitchen by an aged housemaid who had been part of the household since she was thirteen. All four of my grandparents died in their eighties, also in their own beds. Both sets had a daughter, one single the other widowed who, suitably supported by domestic help, were regarded as only doing what was to be expected of them.

When my father died in the third year of my training, my Mother's Mother pointed out that it was my duty to come home. My sisters were teenagers still at school and Mother had good resident help. My brother and I circumvented that one, though not without difficulty - Father had wanted me to complete my training - but the seed was sown - an unmarried daughter's place was at home! Both my sisters married and throughout the war one or the other of them, complete with children, had been at home. Now one was settled in Guildford, the other at Loughton in Essex, my brother lived at Hove. A maid who had been unfortunate enough to produce a baby a year after her husband became a prisoner of war covered the domestic situation for a long time but by degrees we realised that resident domestic help no longer existed and Mother would be alone.

Finally it was decided that Mother would move from East Grinstead to Loughton. We found a house within ten minutes walk of my sister Norah and I would become non-resident. An old gardener who knew the family well remarked gloomily that, 'You can't uproot an old tree' - how right he was. Largely thanks to my sister it worked reasonably well. My mother's generation was probably the last unable to accept that one did have to wash up, peel potatoes and even clean grates. What was yet to materialise was the present day attitude that the alternative is a Home. I was fortunate in having support from both my sisters and my brother. When there is a large age gap in the middle of a family the elder and younger halves tend to view their parents somewhat differently. My brothers and I had always regarded the younger two as children and I found my youngest sister's 'Darling Mother' less helpful on the phone than my brother's bracing 'Don't let the old devil get you down'.

'Living out' increased my understanding of all the commuters who scuttled off hoping to be just ahead of the rush hour where one could scarcely find room to stand in the train. I was fortunate too in my friends - Margaret Job (Mrs Crispin) once stayed over night and was found to be a much better nurse that I was!

Non-residence for trained staff was becoming increasingly popular. Knutsford House, next door to the Cavell Home, a block consisting entirely of small self-contained flats, had been built solely for this purpose.

The pressure to reduce the amount of non nursing duties on the nursing staff continued. A ward secretary lightened the Ward Sister's load, but no longer did the Ward Sister do a quick round of the patients with a word for every one of them as she gave out the letters. Similarly as non nursing duties were taken from the student nurse it became more difficult for the beginner to establish friendly relations with her patients. By the time we had sprinkled tea leaves under their beds, swept them up, washed the locker top and dusted the bed rails conversation was no problem. What does one say to a

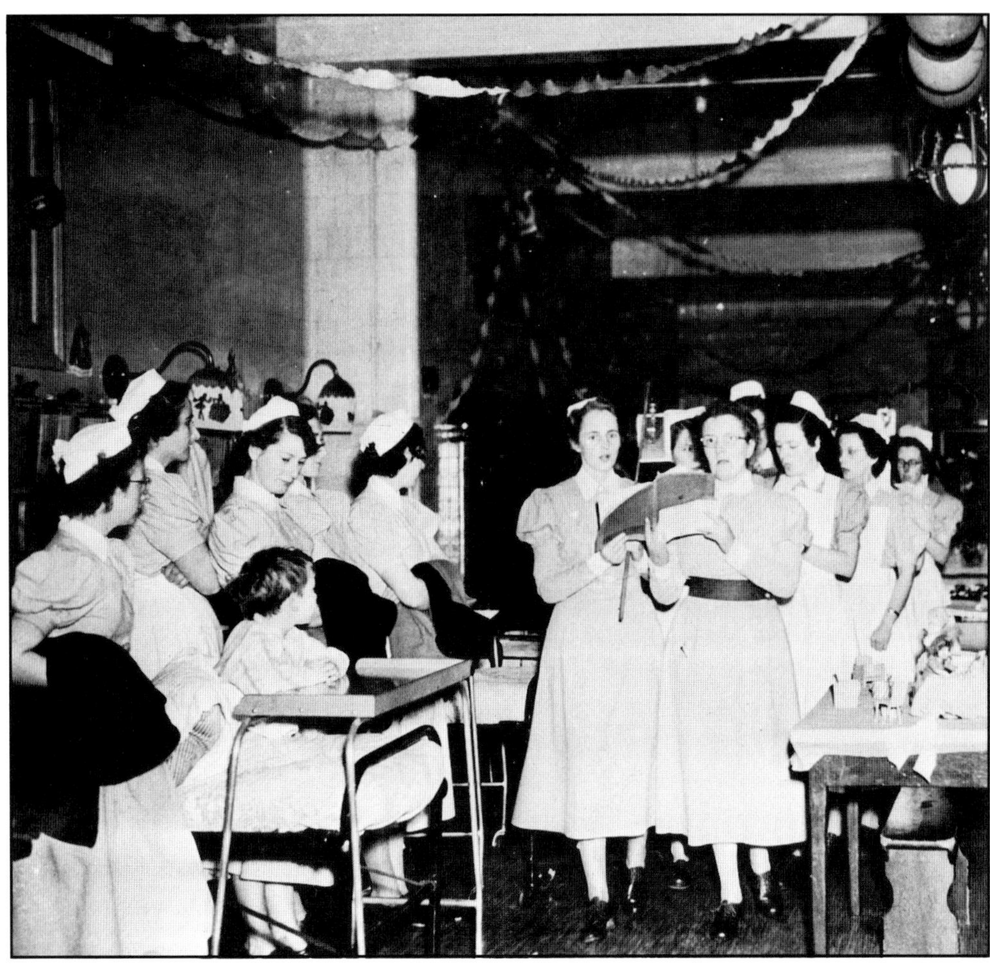

Margaret Broadley and Phyllis Friend lead the Christmas Carols through David Hughes ward.

junior nurse who says, as one did to me, when last I was a patient, that she didn't know what to say to people. Surely that is part of 'the Art of Nursing'.

When first I became a tutor I was all for a Block system and following bad State Examination results in 1939 would have dearly liked to have seen State Finalists given at least a few days in the class room. I was told it was utterly impossible, but the impressive results following my experience at Warley when there was no other way of occupying students convinced me that the Block had much to recommend it. The study Day System had been introduced when I first reached Matron's Office. Seemingly it had been deemed the more expedient method.

Doing the allocation, juggling with bodies like a jigsaw puzzle never quite complete, was to me quite the best job in the hospital. Supervision of the practical side of the nurses training was possibly of greater importance than the academic. I saw the students in the wards so had not completely lost touch with patients. As I got to know the Sisters I learnt that, where the experience was the same, Sister A would encourage the diffident student but Sister B would give the more confident her head. Sister C had an aversion to red hair and titians did badly in her ward, while Sister D positively mothered a girl back from prolonged sick-leave. There was a degree of satisfaction in seeing young people develop - occasionally on prize-giving day even a fond father would comment on it! For all that - twenty years in nurse education and I never did see 'The Block' system at work.

My Mother had a fall, fractured her femur and made a disappointing recovery - finally I accepted that she needed more care than she was receiving and that I must be the one to give it. When Carrie, the manageress of the laundry left, I went quite early in the morning to say goodbye. Beside her desk she had a well stocked table and insisted that I, like all subsequent visitors, had a drink with her - perhaps it was a good way to go. I left at about 4:30 on a Friday afternoon, just as if I was going off for a normal weekend, and caught the train from Whitechapel Station. I thought I didn't mind leaving until I found - to my shame - tears running down my cheeks.

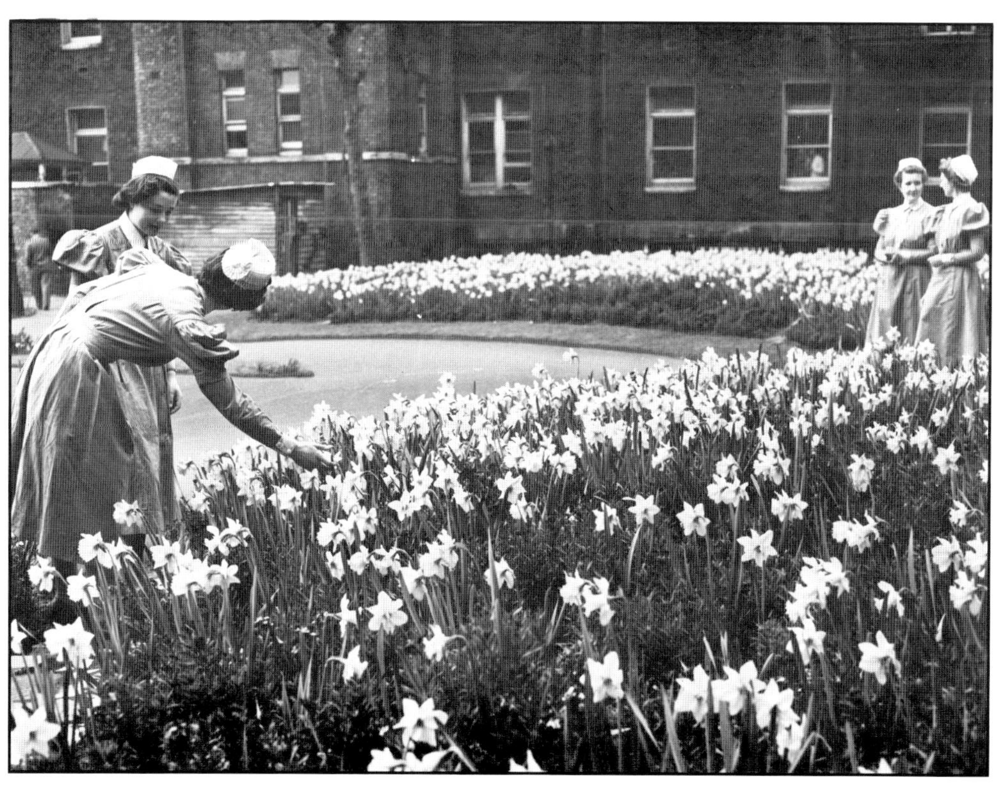

Margaret Broadley and Phyllis Friend admire the hospital garden in spring

CHAPTER FOURTEEN

LIFE BEYOND 'THE LONDON'

Despite my commitments at home, leaving 'The London' did not mean the ending of my involvement with professional nursing and I continued as an Examiner for the General Nursing Council. Thanks to Ceris I was asked to become external examiner to Westminster Hospital's School of Nursing. The regular three or four days I spent there were the highlights of my life, their Nursing Staff, particularly the Matron and Miss Ella Gibbon, the Principal Tutor, were marvellous.

By this time The London Hospital Nurses received their 'hospital certificates' when they had completed their training and became State Registered Nurses. Westminster Hospital still retained as well their own 'Hospital Final Examination'. This included an Examination in Practical Nursing. Every nurse was examined individually in the ward where she was currently working, carrying out treatment pre selected by the candidate, Ward Sister and Tutor. It was the ideal examination setting. The practical part of the General Nursing Council's 'Final State Examination' was held in a classroom where, no matter how well equipped, the bed occupant could be anyone from a convalescent patient borrowed for the occasion to a junior colleague. It was at best an artificial situation. One of Lord Knutsford's favourite stories was of the candidate who, told by the examiner that the patient had just been admitted with a severe head injury, removed his pillows, closed his eyes, crossed his hands on his chest and covered him with a sheet. In response to the examiner's comment that not every head injury dies she replied firmly, 'this one did'.

Examining a nurse on her own ground in a familiar situation is a totally different matter. I always felt that I really could assess the candidate's nursing ability. Every patient in the ward would be willing her to do well and periodically the nearest patient would make an opportunity to tell me just how wonderful Nurse X was. Westminster Hospital, like 'The London' was scattered over several sites covering a wide variety of specialities. I learned something not only from every candidate but from the varied settings.

The examination was held during the candidate's normal working hours - night nurses usually preferred early morning to late evening. 'The London's' Intensive Care Unit had not come into being when I left, so I was first introduced to one at about 6.30 one morning! There were two beds - and two patients. Surveying her equipment my candidate decided there was something missing from the trolley she was about to use. She pointed out that the patients were never left without a nurse but that I should be there whilst she fetched whatever was missing. It was one of the longest two minutes of my life!

Roehampton, one of their annexes, had a 'Burns Unit'. The first time I was there I gathered that the Sister was something of a tartar and the rules on asepsis stringent in the extreme. To my amazement she was one of 'my girls' from the remote past and I could see her hesitating - should the rules be waived - could the soles of MY shoes be regarded as clean. Fortunately I had already got my feet into the footwear my candidate was proffering!

The practical assessment was followed by a brief interview with the candidate. I always tried to introduce something topical, but as every one was likely to ring up the next as I left repetition was tricky. I learnt as much from the interviews as from the practical part. 'Non residence', or living out, for Student Nurses was just beginning. The first time conversation with a candidate revealed that she had a baby, parked in a nearby nursery, I realised how endless was the scope for change.

A retired friend, whom my mother liked, had always come to stay while I was at 'The Westminster'. My next assignment was for one day a week, not too difficult to arrange. Asmall unit, an annexe of a local hospital, wanted a tutor to teach a class of 'pupil nurses'. This was the name given to students taking the two year course of training for enrolment - S.E.N. - State Enrolled Nurse. The intention was sound, the enrolled nurse would be a practical bedside nurse who would fill a valuable place in the ward team, but would not go on to increased responsibility. Pupil Nurse training at The London Hospital did not begin until 1968.

Mine was a small group, English was a second language for practically all of them and they were so anxious to do well. Theirs was a totally different syllabus - needing a different approach. It reminded me of the hymn, 'Tell me the old, old story', surely the writer must have been a teacher - 'Tell me the story slowly, that I may take it in - often, for I forget so soon!' Their practical training was no concern of mine, though I did sometimes give individual instruction in practical nursing in the wards, but with my years of allocation behind me, it seemed that to be training two separate groups in the same wards must be terribly difficult. Admittedly the wards of a general hospital were the only places where the pupil nurse could train, but what a problem for the Ward Sister as well as the administrator.

I put everything I could into that class. What lay ahead of them? They were interested in the care of the sick and anxious to do well. As one of them once confided to me, above all, she would like to be a 'proper nurse' - and State Registration was virtually out of their reach. Years later teaching, at one of the Technical Colleges, State Registered Nurses working for the

Diploma in Nursing, I realised just how much I had gained from that earlier experience.

For the first time my closest associate was a married woman. She and I were the only ones working in the classrooms on a Wednesday afternoon, so our last job was to lock the door and hand the keys in to Matron's Office. Every week she would hand them to me saying 'George will be waiting for me', with the certain knowledge that, even though my mother might be waiting for me, hers was the prior claim. Another lesson learnt.

In the course of time it seemed expedient that I should change from examining for the General Nursing Council's Final Examination for State Registration to that of the Enrolled Nurse. The practical examination for the pupil nurses was, like those at 'Westminster', held in the ward where the pupil was working.

We came across all sorts of unexpected hazards - the examination was essentially an assessment, the candidate showing her practical skills. On one occasion my co-assessor and I arrived at the ward to find that one end had been prepared to resemble as nearly as possible a practical classroom, equipment suitably displayed and a healthy young woman in sensible pyjamas in each bed. The Ward Sister said, 'you can do just what you like with them'. As a mock-up it would have merited high marks! Taking a deep breath I suggested, with a quick look at what were obviously geriatric patients, was there any patient due for, or in need of, attention? On one occasion a candidate asked to change a dressing, enquired, was it a medical or a surgical dressing!

My rudest awakening was at a unit belonging to a famous Teaching Hospital, the Tutor in charge of proceedings regarded the examiners, as one could only assume she regarded her candidates, as of a lower form of animal life. My co-examiner was angry, it is difficult to define what I felt. In some inexplicable way I was allied to the candidates - them and me against the world! - a wholly undesirable frame of mind for an examiner.

By and large, teaching, unlike caring for the sick, does not inspire thanks. On one occasion, at a London Hospital Presentation of Certificates Day, a father, whose second daughter had just completed her training, told me he could not understand why three years of nurse training produced so much more sensible an adult than a similar length of time at a university did, but teaching the less privileged was rewarding. I cherish the memory of the day when on learning her results, one of my pupils rushed out to buy roses - for me!

CHAPTER FIFTEEN

ON TO THE SEVENTIES

As a sixth former, Frances, my sister's only daughter, came back starry eyed from a school visit to an Army Hospital, culminating with tea in an Officer's Mess; from there to The London Hospital's School of Nursing seemed a logical progression. If my advice had been sought I should have advocated Westminster Hospital. It was smaller and I felt their student nurses were under less pressure but, just as my mother had felt the proximity of 'Guys' to London Bridge Station - and East Grinstead trains - made it the obvious choice, my sister thought it would be daft to go further into London, past The London Hospital.

The year was 1970, forty five years since I had watched the 'over thirty' sisters exercise their newly earned right to vote, thirty years since my sister was dismissed for getting married. In the second war casualties had hit the entire population, the carnage among men of the first had not been repeated, though there had been sufficient to ensure a post war stability of nursing staff similar to that of the twenties and thirties. This was no longer the case and, in addition the freedom of women was accelerating.

Frances' and my preparation for nursing were little different. As a Girl Guide I had grown vegetables in an allotment and 'teased' moss reputedly used for surgical dressings. Her Guide experience extended to groups of children, both physically and mentally handicapped and I had arranged for her to accompany the WRVS team on the local 'Meals on Wheels' round, but even there the difference became evident. Fifteen minutes after setting out she was back home - one driver had not turned up, could she borrow the car?

The Princess Alexandra School of Nursing, 'The London's' Nursing School, had been opened in 1967. Incoming sets were no longer isolated at Tredegar House, but started at 'The London' itself. Not all change was for the better - Frances started in the basement of the Lückes Home in a shared room, accommodation previously used exclusively for maids! Conversely, on her first evening she met a school friend who introduced her to a couple of medical students. She went home next evening to collect an evening dress, something I had assured her she would not need for a couple of months. By her first weekend she was dancing at a Ball, with a capital 'B', at 'Guys', for which one of the Medical Students had tickets.

Life in the Nurses' Homes had changed completely. The monthly rental for their rooms was deducted from the students' salary and they paid for every meal as they ate it. They were, in fact, treated as normal adults. It took me four years to complete three years training. Frances may have had two or three days sick leave in three years, certainly she was never warded.

The London's beds were still scattered and Student Nurses were moved round as their experience demanded, all spent three months at the Orthopaedic Unit at Banstead. As we had found, nurses will settle happily anywhere provided they are with their friends. Frances spent her second Christmas at Banstead and, apart from being happy, remembers chiefly how heavy the work was. She was on night duty with a pregnant staff nurse who, rightly, refused to help with the lifting but, wrongly, was not prepared to see that somebody else should.

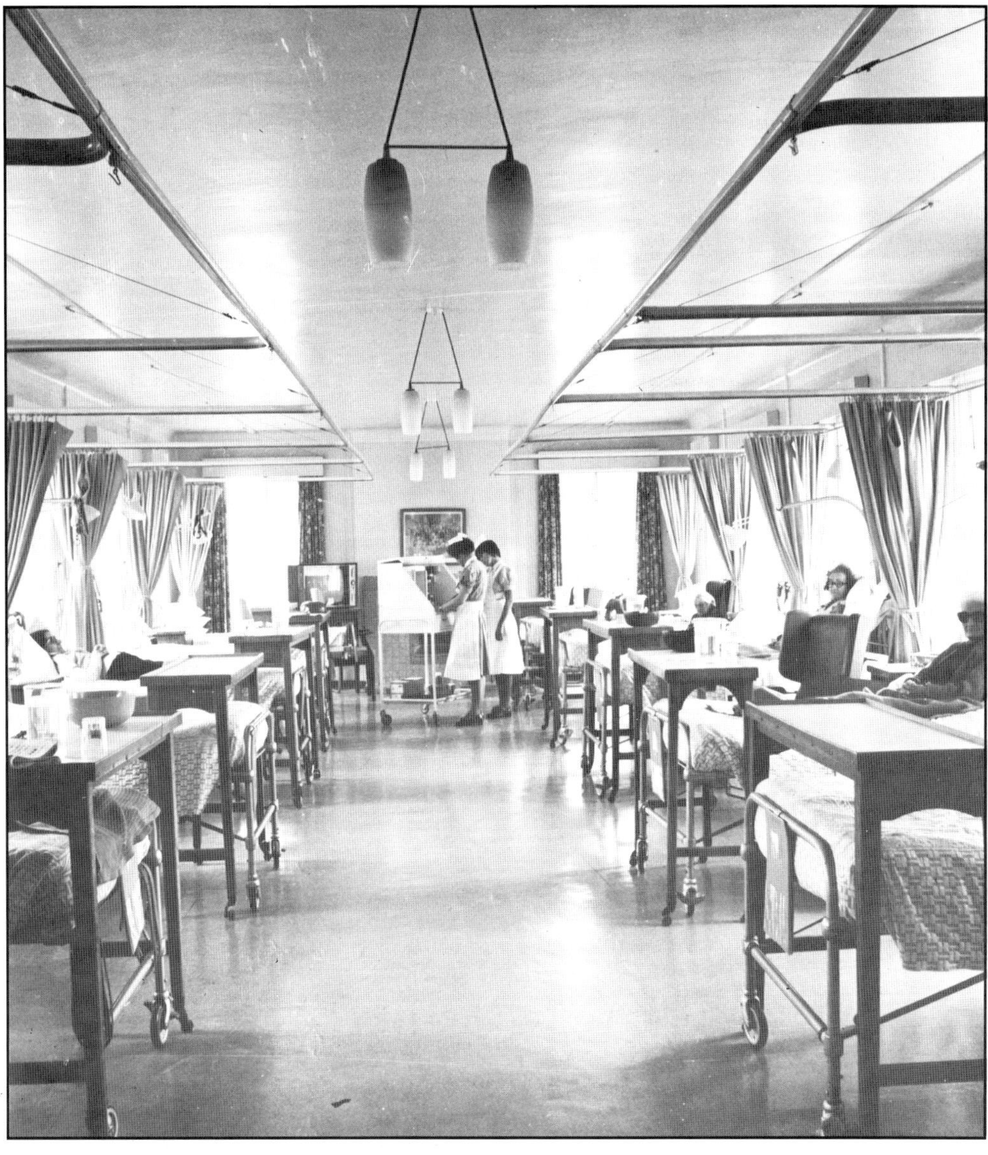

Drug round at Zachery Merton Annexe, Banstead 1977.

Frances' memories of her stay at 'Mile End' are also happy. The wards were terrible and the Nurses' bedrooms overlooked the local cemetery, but it was there that she met Richard, the medical student whom she subsequently married. John Harrison House was a new Nurses' Residence practically next door to the Medical Students Hostel in Whitechapel and on her return from 'Mile End', she was allocated a room there. Every two rooms share a balcony and a bathroom and there are adequate cooking facilities. When Frances was on night duty, Richard had breakfast ready for her when she came off duty!

The dragons, the Sisters of whom we were genuinely terrified, though admitting it was from those that we learnt most, were no more, but the nagging ones, the bullies, persisted in spite of easier conditions. I had met one once and had been pulled up with a jolt by a fatherly patient who comforted me with, 'Don't cry, Nurse, she's not worth it'. The modern generation may be tougher than we were but it still went on. I was horrified to think that one of 'my' Merrymeade girls could have developed into a bully. Where had I gone wrong - ought a Preliminary Course to include treatment of one's juniors? In my case my father advised me - stick to it. Frances' father had been dead for some years and the advice of the eldest of her brothers was the reverse, possibly influenced by the changed position of women. He told her there were plenty of other things she could do - begin again - conflicting advice, but both she and I had won through.

Teaching pupil nurses, I had thought what a problem the inclusion of another set of learners in the ward team must be. To add to the time honoured pattern of State Registered Staff Nurses (S.R.N.) first, second and third year students, first and second year pupils **AND** an Enrolled Nurse (S.E.N.) must have needed the wisdom of Solomon. From Frances and her friends, I gathered that the established S.E.N. could be a blessing to a junior student, but for the student nearing the end of her third year, the newly qualified S.E.N., whose total experience was less than her own, was difficult to take. Which of them was the senior? It must also have been difficult to find posts within the hospital for the S.E.N. The London Hospital Pupil Nurse School was closed in 1984.

Financially, the position of the student nurse of the seventies was totally different from that of the pre war probationer, whose salary rose from £30 to £40 a year, paid quarterly, by the end of her training. Most student nurses had banking accounts, but how could any seemingly intelligent woman open a joint account with an impecunious young man with whom there was no legal commitment - but it happened.

I saw a certain amount of medical students too - the relationship of doctors and nurses had subtly changed over the years. How much had the universal use of Christian names influenced this? We had been brought up to see doctors as being far more heavily worked than we were - there was consideration as well as respect. 'You'll see those boys don't go hungry to bed' was my Ward Sister's instruction to me after a late night delivery my first night as night probationer in a maternity ward. The housemen of my probationer years were war veterans, towards whom the Nursing Staff had a protective attitude. They were of course older than usual and we for our own part had reason to remember the war. Their leaving parties were apt to be more riotous than is generally considered suitable but the night Nursing Staff gave the sort of loyalty one finds among brothers and sisters - although we did not know it I suspect the Night Sisters felt the same! I was therefore somewhat surprised when a young houseman, I cannot imagine how I came to be left to entertain him, told me that he didn't mind checking drugs with a nurse to help out but he resented being given the key of the Drug Cupboard.

It is seventy years since I worked in that maternity ward. 'Sister Vic' as she was affectionately known, a shortening of the name of the sub-ward, would have been aware if her S.R.A. or J.R.A., senior or junior resident accoucheur, had not been to bed for 48 hours - and she would have done something about it. The Sister today is younger, presumably relationship of doctor and nurse have changed if he, or she, no longer merits the compassion given to the patient. Surely Sister - or Charge Nurse - should be aware of the plight of the hapless houseman?

All things considered, training in the seventies produced well balanced capable young women. There was one great difference, for the first time this century there had been no major war claiming men's lives. The surplus woman had ceased to exist. Not only did increased freedom give every woman a much wider choice of career but, working far harder than ever her mother did, she expects to combine home, family and career throughout her working life.

CHAPTER SIXTEEN

SPANNING SEVENTY YEARS

These things shall be! A loftier race
Than ere the world has seen shall rise,
With flame of freedom in their souls,
And light of knowledge in their eyes.
John Addinton Symonds.
(1840 - 1893)

In 1986 I was to be admitted to 'The London' for heart surgery. The phone rang at mid-day on a Saturday, a call from 'The London', why had I not arrived. The voice at the other end accepted that this was the first I had heard of it and the deadline was extended - be there by 4pm! I had been told that sometimes very little notice of admission was given so I was vaguely ready, even though there was a half roasted chicken in the oven! Duly reporting as requested I was somewhat daunted to be told I must have made a mistake, there was no bed. A voice off suggested, 'She's on the list for Monday.' After some delay, I joined the other patients in the day room for supper - one by one the meals were dished out and finally a sandwich was plonked down in front of me with the information that that was all that was left - the remark, 'and I hope it chokes you', didn't follow, probably I just felt it was implied - after all, I had had no lunch - or tea! However, that was the moment of truth, the moment when I learned that in the hospital setting of the late twentieth century, it is one's fellow patients that matter. It was suggested I found out what was in the sandwich and, from their own stores, I was offered butter - cheese and jam! They really cared.

In fairness to 'The London' I must say that my subsequent care was excellent - 'black Saturday' was just unfortunate and my adverse criticism ends with it.

The modern patient is on a conveyor belt, from Theatre to Intensive Care Unit is the first stage. The art of nursing changes but is there. At every stage, apparently effortlessly, my toothbrush, spectacles, hearing aid and watch were there when I wanted them. It is one of the regrets of my life that I have no recollection of Intensive Care. Next came a high dependency unit. I looked round hopefully and wondered what I was doing with those ill people, it must be a mistake. I enquired of a passing nurse, when would the newspaper man be round and was told, loftily, that no newspapers were allowed; I was more than ever convinced that it was a mistake. However, time passed and a couple of days later a staff nurse inserted me into my dressing gown and slippers, took me firmly by the arm and walked me back to the general ward. That was where life began again.

It takes time to grasp that today's patient, so far from being confined to bed, is free to roam not only in his own ward but throughout the hospital. He wanders down to buy something from the shop or use the public telephone. One of my fellow patients was the husband of a friend of a neighbour of mine. He and I spent a morning discussing if one decided to abscond, how long would it be before one was missed? Patients not only wandered, but were dispatched in wheel chairs to all sorts of destinations. In the X-ray Dept there was the same camaraderie as existed in the ward. The second time a man I thought looked too ill to be out of his bed cheered me up with a funny story, of his fellow patients, it dawned on me that he probably thought of me much as I did of him. Ward routine was minimal, 'eight o'clock lights out' had long been gone, but I was surprised to find a fellow patient sitting quietly on a chair beside his bed, reading the paper - at 2 o'clock in the morning! The daily visiting time was more like an invasion, whole families would descend on their relative, dumping the baby on Grannie's bed, they would remain solidly until the bell indicating 'time' rang.

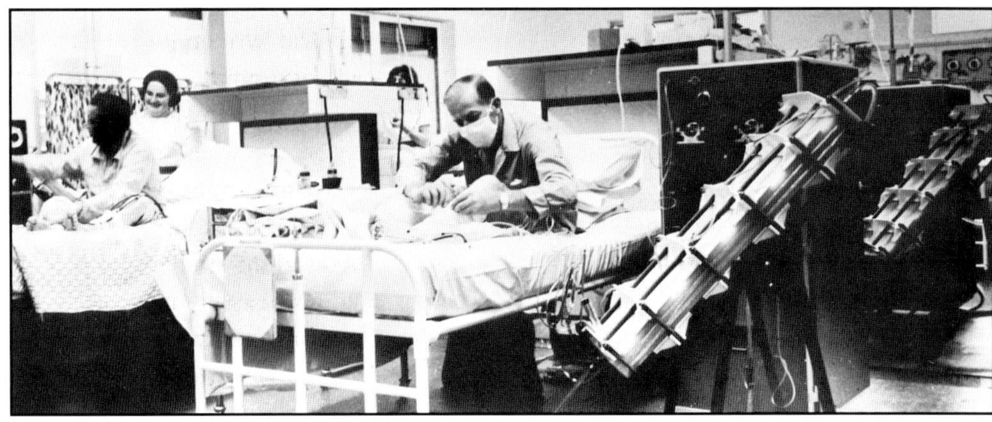

Dialysis Unit, Hanbury ward.

Supervision of nursing students has perforce always been unobtrusive, but I was somewhat taken aback when a student nurse, bearing down upon me with a dressing trolley, informed me that he could not be expected to know how to do something he had never done before! As he was about to replace a dressing and bandage, no longer necessary, with an elastic stocking, I was somewhat at a loss as to my role - confidante, tutor or patient?

It was at this stage that I encountered Fiona, a granddaughter of my cousin Harold, father of the baby my mother and sister had taken over during the blitz. Harold and I had always been friends, I had seen his children grow up and now and again had met his daughter's children. I knew that Fiona had applied to 'The London' for training, but it was most unexpected when, working in a nearby ward, she casually blew in to see me! A couple of days later she announced that her grandparents were staying with her parents in Hertfordshire and she would bring them to see me. Never, in all my years at 'The London' had Harold done that. It was finally only Harold she brought, bearing what Fiona considered suitable reading material. He said she had told him a book was much better than flowers as he had intended. In the course of his visit he assured me that Fiona was a 'grand girl' - a good description.

Half way through the following Sunday morning one of my nurses informed me that I had a visitor, a man in a dressing gown. Nothing in hospital is surprising, but I thought it was probably someone from Loughton, but I'd never seen him before. He told me he was a stranger to London, had been admitted as an emergency and was waiting for heart surgery. I had a feeling that I knew what was coming - he had told one of the nurses of his fears - I would have liked to know just what Fiona had said to him!

Not long after my father's death, towards the end of my third year, on another Sunday morning, my ward sister retired to her room for a cup of coffee commending to my special care a dying patient. I found that her saline rectal drip had come adrift and was dripping in to her bed, to lessen her discomfort I switched it off, saw that she was warm and dry - and proceeded to dismantle the apparatus. On her return, Sister was scathing! A consultant had ordered the treatment - a houseman had 'written it up' - she herself had got it going - and I - a mere probationer...........! Towards the end of her diatribe, she went on, 'I'm not saying it wasn't the right thing to do but you were not the right person to do it'. As I showed the stranger my scar and calmed his fears my mind went back sixty years to that incident - sixty years and a whole world apart! Each instance involved plain common sense. My generation prided themselves that they knew the idiosyncrasies of every patient, it was their physical, rather than mental, condition in which we were involved. The girl of the eighties thought of the patient as a whole and was not, as we were, afraid of the powers that be nor bound by petty convention. She concentrated on the essentials.

I had one further encounter with Fiona - the nurse. She rang me up some months later. Her grandparents were again staying at her home. She would drive to Much Hadham via Loughton and take me to see them. She came, with a mufti coat thrown over her uniform dress, and, still wearing it, made tea for us all on our arrival. My mind again went back sixty years - I had been summoned to Matron's Office - I had been seen crossing the hospital garden, in Outdoor Uniform, wearing only one glove!!

From my hospital bed, I remembered my first medical ward, in the early twenties. In one of the cardiac beds was a stout middle aged woman, Mrs Leakey, diagnosed as 'heart failure'. Oedematous and short of breath, the ubiquitous water pillow under the draw sheet, she was propped up by a back rest and pillows. How did her lot compare with mine? The ward, heated by a coal fire, was regulated, quiet, clean and cold. No TV, no radio, lights out at eight o'clock every night, visiting times were one hour on Wednesday afternoons, one and a half on Saturdays and two on Sundays, two visitors at a time only and no children under twelve.

Confined to bed, like the majority of patients, Mrs Leakey's nursing care lacked nothing. Suitably fed, her fluid intake and output meticulously recorded, probably T.L.C. (Tender loving care) was the most important part of her treatment. How much thought was given to her as a person, was she lonely, bored, apprehensive? No NHS safety net, almoners, social or ancillary workers, all these services were represented by the Ward Sister, the patients' counsellor, advisor and friend.

Since then, women have, first, been given the vote and later, were able to work after marriage. The age of entry to nursing has dropped to eighteen - Florence Nightingale set it at twenty five. State Registration is mandatory. The fourth, staff, year no longer compulsory, three years completes the contract. Two major wars within fifty years have ensured slow turnover of trained staff. The long-standing ward sisters of the 20s and 30s, from whom my generation gained so much, should have been the mothers and grandmothers of the leaders of the country today. The carnage of the second was less and more widely spread, but sufficient to produce stability of trained staff for the 40s and 50s.

Care of the sick has changed with medical advances and the nurse requires new technical skills. Nurse training has been adapted to provide the requisite technical knowledge but the student still needs to learn the practical art. In the twenties it was said that if one was not learning one was teaching. Frances' generation summed it up as 'see one - do one - teach one'! No longer is it a man's world, more and more barriers have been lifted. The able young woman of today is aware that anything man can do so too can she. Nursing has to compete with every known profession for the services of right minded girls - and boys. Care of the sick has a certain pull but the girl of today knows she can become a judge, an astronaut, even Prime Minister AND marry and have a family.

Just as the pictures of wartime training are provided by the people involved, it is the nurse of today who can throw some light on the present.

Fiona Courtauld (nee Hadlee) writes,

I have always been fascinated by illness and hospitals, but when I returned from a year's travel in South East Asia I really had no idea of what to expect from my nurse's training.

I think all of us in the May 1985 intake at 'The London', most of us in our early twenties with some experience of other occupations, were shocked by the physical and mental demands of our initial training; made all the more exhausting by active social lives.

The majority of us accepted the offer of nurses accommodation at the hospital, but I moved out within two months and by the end of the first year most of my fellow students had followed suit. Our independent external lives probably made the hard work all the more arduous. 30 % of the students did not complete the three year training, all opting for completely different careers.

One fifth of the intake for our set was male, but this ratio was not to last - only two men were finally to qualify! I, personally, never seriously considered giving up. The psychiatric block of my training was my particular low point because the patients were so thoroughly institutionalised and, in the short time we were with them, never seemed to improve. Whether care in the community is a better answer, I do not know.

On arrival in the wards I was amazed at the youth of the staff and how very much responsibility they were given. For some reason I had expected to be under the watchful eye of an, at least, middle-aged sister.

Over the three years we were exposed to most medical and surgical wards; theatres, midwifery, paediatrics, accident and care of the elderly and outpatients, but one got little managerial experience; this to come only on qualification.

The theoretical instruction was relevant, but owing to staff shortage, clinical practice was not always adequately demonstrated or supervised, such as the administration of drugs.

In the second year of my training the drug policy changed, a single qualified staff nurse being now all that was required to dispense the drugs. Student participation in this obviously declined, reducing an important learning opportunity.

The majority of the nursing staff were female and unmarried. After job cuts were introduced many of the staff posts were frozen, students completing their training were not guaranteed jobs, and loyalty and morale sank. A surprising number of my peers and friends moved to other hospitals and training colleges e.g. midwifery, but I felt privileged to have been offered a job and in due course joined the Renal Unit.

Throughout training, one's practical experience had been sheltered, there had been little opportunity to shoulder responsibility. Overnight, on qualifying, one was given a daunting amount of responsibility, one's role totally altered, staff shortages exaggerated this.

The Renal Unit was highly specialised so the new managerial responsibility coupled with the scarcity of other knowledgeable Renal specialists and the concurrent demand on one's time meant that it was an exceptionally challenging post which I thoroughly enjoyed. Although it was hard, one learnt an enormous amount very quickly, working under an exceptionally knowledgeable, conscientious and supportive team.

During my time at 'The London', finance and budgeting became real issues. Probably all students are less conscious of this side of hospital care, but as a staff nurse I was acutely aware of the day to day ward finances and the ramifications of national politics.

Agency nurses were an increasing preoccupation in the late 1980s. A 'Reed Nursing Agency' was established in 'The London' itself! On night duty particularly agency nurses predominated. This considerable expense made the freezing of permanent posts, the loss of promising students to other hospitals and other cuts all the harder to understand.

Possibly because of poor pay and bad press about nursing as a career, fewer and fewer applications for training were received by the nursing college. Some of the more recent students did not speak English as a first language and communication at times could be a problem. This was also true of the patients, a number of the local Bengali population, particularly women, could not speak English at all, which obviously made the provision of proper care difficult.

Visiting hours became more relaxed, open from 2 - 8pm; this in many ways had advantages, but the ward was always full of people which gave the patient less time to recuperate.

The pace of patients being admitted and discharged seemed to accelerate over the years. It was not unusual for several people to be discharged late on Friday evening due to the urgent requirements of beds, without much consideration for whether they had food at home or easy transport. One might have two days off duty and only recognise 50% of the patients on one's return.

The training I had undergone emphasised the needs of the person as a 'whole' inclusive of his/her family and religion. The importance of information flow as a two way process from patient to nurse and nurse to patient was crucial.

My time spent at 'The London' was an incredibly rewarding and happy time, exciting, exhilarating and exhausting, but now I have a family of my own, I understand the difficulties of returning to hospital nursing though it certainly held me in good stead for the sleepless nights!"

Since then nurses have campaigned for parity with university students seemingly ignoring their need to gain practical nursing skills.

Another development, the growth of day case surgery, increases the difficulty of learning these skills. It is estimated that one in four of all surgical procedures are now carried out on this basis. These are the patients, previously in hospital for about two weeks, who formed the bulk of 'comfortably ill patients' on whom we all learnt. The methods vary a little. The patients are selected with care and in many cases a district nurse is involved both before and after surgery. Two of my friends have recently undergone such surgery to their complete satisfaction, it must however, increase the pressure on hospital nursing staff.

Two hundred and fifty years ago, the term used to describe the sick man was 'miserable object', today he is 'the client' or even 'the customer'! Inevitably, change will continue, the nurse of tomorrow will probably lift and turn the 'patient' by the flick of a switch. Was the patient of say fifty years ago better treated in hospital than he is today? Physically he was more comfortable, his physical well being was paramount, but, for myself, I would choose today.In the modern hospital, highly sophisticated techniques, assisted by modern drugs, produce evermore remarkable results. In this setting, 'the patient', unless he reaches hospital in an unconscious state, is an essential member of the team - it is his life that is involved.

Fifty years ago, when the Health Service was new, the patient was not the arbiter of his fate. After a couple of weeks in hospital, particularly following surgery, he would be sent into the country for a couple of weeks convalescence. Was that necessarily the best thing for women, with children whose family could not afford to visit?

The running of a ward today is not as meticulous as it was then, but the ward is a more homely place and the sick man remains in close contact with his family and friends. The 'patient' is not a 'hip' or a 'heart'. What is being done is in his individual interest and with his consent. If on leaving hospital he is to walk a mile a day his family are aware of this - and will see that he does so.

Day care treatment closely involves the sick man's family. How much better for him to recover in his own home, sleeping in his own bed. It is difficult to visualise the hospital of tomorrow. Increasingly Hospices will give loving care to both the terminally ill and their families. Special provision may be needed, as the numbers of centenarians grows, for those of extreme old age, but that again would not be in hospital.

One of the major challenges now facing the nursing profession is the concept of the patient as a whole person. The student nurse of today, with less experience of bedside care, sees him in this light with a family and background much more clearly than her predecessors have done. This surely is the basic principle of the Art of Nursing